CARDIAC ANAESTHESIA: PROBLEMS AND INNOVATIONS

DEVELOPMENTS IN CRITICAL CARE MEDICINE AND ANESTHESIOLOGY

Prakash, O. (ed.): Applied Physiology in Clinical Respiratory Care. 1982. ISBN 90-247-2662-X.

McGeown, Mary G.: Clinical Management of Electrolyte Disorders. 1983. ISBN 0-89838-559-8.

Scheck, P.A., Sjöstrand, U.H., and Smith, R.B. (eds.): Perspectives in High Frequency Ventilation. 1983. ISBN 0-89838-571-7.

Stanley, T.H., and Petty, W.C. (eds.): New Anesthetic Agents, Devices and Monitoring Techniques. 1983. ISBN 0-89838-566-0.

Prakash, O. (ed.): Computing in Anesthesia and Intensive Care. 1983. ISBN 0-89838-602-0.

Stanley, T.H., and Petty, W.C. (eds.): Anesthesia and the Cardiovascular System. 1984. ISBN 0-89838-626-8.

Van Kleef, J.W., Burm, A.G.L., and Spierdijk, J. (eds.): Current Concepts in Regional Anaesthesia. 1984. ISBN 0-89838-644-6.

Prakash, O. (ed.): Critical Care of the Child. 1984. ISBN 0-89838-661-6.

Stanley, T.H., and Petty, W.C. (eds.): Anesthesiology: Today and Tomorrow. 1985. ISBN 0-89838-705-1.

Rahn, H., and Prakash, O. (eds.): Acid-base Regulation and Body Temperature. 1985. ISBN 0-89838-708-6.

Stanley, T.H., and Petty, W.C. (eds.): Anesthesiology 1986. 1986. ISBN 0-89838-779-5.

de Lange, S., Hennis, P.J., and Kettler, D. (eds.): Cardiac Anaesthesia: Problems and Innovations. 1986. ISBN 0-89838-794-9.

CARDIAC ANAESTHESIA: PROBLEMS AND INNOVATIONS

edited by

S. DE LANGE, P.J. HENNIS

Department of Anaesthesiology
Leiden University Hospital, Leiden
The Netherlands

and

D. KETTLER

Georg-August-Universität, Göttingen
Federal Republic of Germany

1986 **MARTINUS NIJHOFF PUBLISHERS**
a member of the KLUWER ACADEMIC PUBLISHERS GROUP
DORDRECHT / BOSTON / LANCASTER

Distributors

for the United States and Canada: Kluwer Academic Publishers, 190 Old Derby Street, Hingham, MA 02043, USA
for the UK and Ireland: Kluwer Academic Publishers, MTP Press Limited, Falcon House, Queen Square, Lancaster LA1 1RN, UK
for all other countries: Kluwer Academic Publishers Group, Distribution Center, P.O. Box 322, 3300 AH Dordrecht, The Netherlands

Library of Congress Cataloging in Publication Data

Cardiac anaesthesia.

(Developments in critical care medicine and anaesthesiology)
Based on a Boerhaave symposium entitled "Recent advances in cardiac anaesthesia," held May 9-10, 1985 in Leiden, Netherlands; organized by the Faculty of Medicine, University of Leiden.
Includes bibliographies and index.
1. Anesthesia in cardiology--Congresses. 2. Heart--Surgery--Congresses. 2. Heart--Surgery--Congresses. I. Lange, S. de. II. Hennis, P. J. III. Kettler, Dietrich. IV. Rijksuniversiteit te Leiden. Faculteit der Geneeskunde. [DNLM: 1. Anesthesiology--congresses. 2. Heart--drug effects--congresses. 3. Monitoring, Physiologic--congresses. WG 460 C2675 1985]
RD87.3.H43 1986 617'.967412 86-856
ISBN 0-89838-794-9

ISBN 0-89838-794-9 (this volume)

Book information

This publication is based upon a Boerhaave Symposium, organized by the Faculty of Medicine, University of Leiden.

Copyright

PRINTED IN THE NETHERLANDS

PREFACE

In the past decade there has been a spectacular increase in the number of open heart operations performed. This is largely due to the increased demand for coronary artery bypass grafting procedures. In response, cardiac anaesthesiologists have had to adapt established anaesthetic techniques and also develop new ones in order to provide safe and stress free anaesthesia for this type of surgery. Advances in diagnostic techniques and monitoring have made a great impact on these developments.

In Europe, different centres have evolved various new anaesthetic and monitoring techniques to meet this challenge. Unfortunately, national and language barriers have resulted in a relatively low information exchange between these centres. In contrast, national meetings in the United States ensure that their cardiac anaesthesiologists are promptly informed about new developments.

A symposium entitled: "Recent Advances in Cardiac Anaesthesia" was held on May 9-10, 1985 in Leiden, The Netherlands, in order to to rectify this situation so that there would also be a free exchange of new ideas and methods in Europe. This book contains the papers presented at this meeting. In addition to the problems and innovations of cardiac anaesthesia and monitoring that were discussed, it was also proposed that these meetings should be held annually in different European countries under the guidance of an informal work group of cardiac anaesthesiologists. With this purpose in mind, the European Association of Cardiothoracic Anaesthesiologists was formed during the symposium.

Simon de Lange

TABLE OF CONTENTS

CONTRIBUTORS

Dr. B. Amari
III Servizio di Anestesia e Rianimazione
Centro A. De Gasperis
Ente Ospedaliero Cà Granda-Niguarda
Milano 20162
Italy

Dr. J.G. Bovill
Afdeling Anaesthesiologie
Academisch Ziekenhuis Leiden
Rijnsburgerweg 10
2333 AA Leiden
The Netherlands

Dr. N.P. de Bruijn
Department of Anesthesiology
Duke University Medical Center
Durham, North Carolina 27710
U.S.A.

Dr. A.V.G. Bruschke
Afdeling Cardiologie
Academisch Ziekenhuis Leiden
Rijnsburgerweg 10
2333 AA Leiden
The Netherlands

Dr. W. Haider
Klinik für Anästhesia
der Universität Wien
Spitalgasse 23
1090 Wien
Austria

Dr. G. Hempelman
Abteilung für Anaesthesiologie und Intensivmedizin
des Klinikums der Justus-Liebig Universität
Klinikstrasse 29
D-6300 Giessen, F.R.G.

Dr. P.J. Hennis
Afdeling Anaesthesiologie
Academisch Ziekenhuis Leiden
Rijnsburgerweg 10
2333 AA Leiden
The Netherlands

Dr. C.C. Hug Jr.
Department of Anesthesiology
Emory University Clinic
1365 Clifton Road NE
Atlanta, Georgia 30322
U.S.A.

Dr. G.F. Karliczek
Afdeling Anaesthesiology
Academisch Ziekenhuis Groningen
Oostersingel 59
9713 EZ Groningen
The Netherlands

Dr. D. Kettler
Georg-August-Universität
Robert Koch Strasse 40
D-3400 Göttingen, F.R.G.

Dr. S. de Lange
Afdeling Anaesthesiologie
Academisch Ziekenhuis Leiden
Rijnsburgerweg 10
2333 AA Leiden
The Netherlands

Dr. S. Reiz
Department of Anaesthesia
University Hospital
90185 Umea
Sweden

Dr. J.A. Richter
Deutsches Herzcentrum München
Lothstrasse 11
8000 München 2, F.R.G.

Dr. G. Settergren
Department of Anaesthesia
Karolinska Hospital
Box 60500
S-104 01 Stockholm
Sweden

Dr. H. Sonntag
Georg-August-Universität
Robert Koch Strasse 40
D-3400 Göttingen, F.R.G.

Dr. T.H. Stanley
Department of Anesthesiology
School of Medicine/Medical Center
50 North Medical Drive
Salt Lake City, Utah 84132
USA

Dr. P.J.A. van der Starre
Medisch Centrum de Klokkenberg
Galderseweg 81
4836 AE Breda
The Netherlands

WHAT SHOULD THE CARDIAC ANAESTHESIOLOGIST KNOW ABOUT HEART CATHETERIZATION?

A.V.G. Bruschke

There are two situations in which an anaesthesiologist will be interested in catheterization data, namely when a patient with significant heart disease has to undergo major non-cardiac surgery and when a patient has to undergo heart surgery. In both instances the anaesthesiologist should have a good understanding of the patient's hemodynamic situation which should enable him to anticipate and possibly avoid cardiac complications. The situation is more complex in cardiac surgery than it is in non-cardiac surgery since a heart operation itself may totally change the patient's hemodynamic status. Therefore, the cardiac anaesthesiologist should not only be able to interpret accurable pre-operative data but he should also be aware of changes caused by the surgical intervention. Catheterization data are extremely valuable and often indispensable in the evaluation of cardiac patients but care should be taken to interpret these data within the context of a complete clinical evaluation. Obviously it is impossible to review all aspects of cardiac catheterization here. We will just try to highlight some general principles and aspects that appear to be regularly overlooked.

In a catheterization laboratory generally the following techniques are performed:

1. Angiography
2. Hemodynamic studies
3. Special studies and function tests, such as:
    - Pacing
    - Metabolic tests
    - Electrophysiologic studies
    - Spasm provocative tests
4. Interventions, such as:
    - Pacemaker insertion
    - Thrombolysis
    - Percutaneous transluminal coronary angioplasty

1. <u>Angiography</u>

In most catheterization laboratories currently emphasis is placed on angiographic studies. In fact, in many centers patients with ischemic heart disease, are studied only by coronary and left ventricular angiography. The low morbidity and mortality of coronary surgery appear to testify that this

is a sound and practical approach. One should realize, however, that a coronary arteriogram, despite recent technical improvements, has certain diagnostic limitations. This concerns mainly the estimation of narrowings. Generally narrowings are expressed as percentage reduction of lumen diameter but occasionally it is impossible to be certain of the original diameter of the vessel. This is particularly the case in diffusely diseased vessels. Eccentric and highly irregular lesions may also present problems. In such cases sometimes the estimation of narrowing is based upon the projection in which the narrowing produces the greatest reduction of lumen diameter but this may easily lead to overestimation of the severity of such lesions. Unfortunately there is no method to overcome this problem. Even sophisticated computerized measuring devices are of limited value in this respect.
Another source of error may be the presence or absence of collateral flow. If a severely narrowed but not occluded vessel receives collaterals from another artery this does not mean that the myocardium is sufficiently protected if this vessel becomes occluded since the coronary arteriogram hardly presents an indication as to the potential flow through the collaterals. Conversely, if no collaterals are seen this does not mean that no collateral pathways are present. This is sometimes nicely illustrated in patients with coronary arterial spasm in whom collateral channels may appear and disappear according to the degree of narrowing caused by changes in vasal tone. The situation is only slightly different if an artery is occluded. In such cases the absence of collaterals is usually seen in conjunction with left ventricular scar tissue but the presence of collaterals, even if the occluded vessel is angiographically well opacified, does not rule out the possibility of severe residual ischemia. These factors should be realized when a patient is considered for surgery or a surgical procedure is planned. Special attention deserves the presence of stenosis of the left main coronary artery. This is considered such an ominous prognostic sign that in practically all clinical trials on medical versus surgical treatment of coronary artery disease such patients are excluded from randomization. This may be justified but it has not been proven that the prognosis of "left main disease" is significantly worse as compared to the prognosis of "three vessel disease". In fact, in the Cleveland Clinic series (1) the natural history of both conditions appeared to be almost the same. Five-year survival was 51% in the first and 47% in the second category and 10-year survival was also practically the same in both groups. It may therefore be argued that 3-vessel disease represents the same stringent indication for surgery as does left main disease.

2. Hemodynamic studies

2.1. Cardiac output

In hemodynamic studies cardiac output, from which stroke volume is easily derived, is one of the most essential data.

Cardiac output can be calculated by:

1. Fick method
2. Indication dilation methods
   Dye dilution
   Thermodilution
3. Angiographic methods
4. Conductance catheter method

Of the various methods te Fick method, if properly performed, is still the most reliable and is often used as gold standard to evaluate other methods. The principle is simple: oxygen consumption and arterial and venous oxygen content are determined and from these values it is calculated how much blood must have passed the lungs to transport the oxygen consumed. The following formula is used:

$$\text{Cardiac output} = \frac{\text{Ox. consumption}}{\text{arterial-venous Ox. difference}}$$

Of course, by this method pulmonary flow is determined which only equals cardiac output in the absence of intracardiac shunts.
Measuring oxygen consumption is somewhat cumbersome and therefore indicator dilution methods are frequently used. Among these thermodilution has the advantage of easy repeatability without prohibitive accumulation of dye. This method, which has an acceptable accuracy, is also very suitable for postoperative monitoring of cardiac output.
Angiographic methods employ left ventricular enddiastolic and systolic outlines from which left ventricular volumes and stroke volume (diastolic volume minus systolic volume) are calculated. If multiplied by heart rate cardiac output is obtained. Stroke volume thus determined represents total stroke volume whereas by the previously mentioned methods effective stroke volume is calculated. If no valvular insufficiency or intracardiac shunt is present total stroke volume is the same as effective stroke volume. In the presence of aortic or mitral valve regurgitation effective stroke volume equals total stroke volume minus regurgitant volume. Therefore, in the case of valvular insufficiency regurgitant volume may be assessed by determining both total and effective stroke volume.
A promising device to measure stroke volume is the conductance catheter which was developed in Leiden (2). This method employs eight electrodes that are equally spaced near the far end of a catheter positioned along the left ventricular axis. A 20 kHz current is applied between electrodes 1 and 8 and from the voltage between adjacent electrodes electrical conductance in the left ventricular cavity is determined by which left ventricular volume can be calculated. This method allows continuous measurement of left ventricular volume and pressure and has the additional advantage that the hemodynamic situation is undisturbed by injection of contrast medium. Its accuracy seems adequate but has to be further verified in a variety of conditions.

2.2 Valve areas

Cardiac output is the cornerstone in calculating areas of stenotic valves. The general formula for valve areas is:

$$\text{Area} = K \frac{\text{Flow}}{44.5 \sqrt{\Delta P}}$$

In the formula K is a constant which has a specific value for each valve location. Flow is the flow across the valve during the period the valve is open, that is during diastole in mitral valve calculations and during systole in aortic valve calculations. The mean pressure gradient across the valve (Δ P) also relates to the period the valve is open. The formula shows that accurate measurement of cardiac output, from which Flow is derived, is critically important in determining valvular areas in a reliable manner. To a certain extent cardiac output is more important than the pressure gradient since the calculated area is proportional to the first and a square root function of the second parameter. Calculations are unreliable if the stenotic valve is also insufficient. If this is the case then the flow across the valve is no longer directly related to effective cardiac output because of the to and fro movement of the regurgitant volume. This, however, concerns only the insufficient valve. Aortic regurgitation, for instance, does not preclude reliable calculation of mitral valve area.

2.3 Assessment of myocardial function

One of the most challenging but at the same time the most difficult task of an invasive cardiologist is to evaluate myocardial function. Studies on myocardial function usually deal primarily with left ventricular pump function. This is not illogical because in most situations left ventricular function is more critical than right ventricular function. However, the reverse is occasionally true, for instance in right ventricular myocardial infarction. Most left ventricular function parameters deal with global pump function. In this concept no attention is paid to the fact that particularly in ischemic heart disease important differences between various portions of the heart muscle may exist to the extent that some portions may be hyperkinetic whereas other portions do not contract at all or even bulge out during systole. It may be argued that this is of limited importance because the hemodynamic situation is determined by total left ventricular function. Perhaps this is true in the untreated patient but the situation is entirely different if one tries to predict the outcome of interventions, particularly that of surgery. In a surgical candidate with poor left ventricular function the prognosis is clearly related to the residual amount of relatively normal myocardium which is only partly reflected by total pump function indices. With these restrictions in mind we will now briefly review some commonly used parameters.

2.3.1. Left ventricular end-diastolic pressure and cardiac output

Left ventricular end-diastolic pressure is often assumed to represent left ventricular preload. Although this is not unconditionally true it is a reasonable assumption for practical purposes. According to Starling's law, stroke volume is related to preload. Stroke volume rises as a function of preload up to a point where the curve bends downward but this point is probably never reached in clinical conditions. Due to the interrelationship of stroke-volume and preload these parameters should always be considered together. Even then, however, they yield limited information about left ventricular pump function. Left ventricular end-diastolic pressure is determined by a variety of factors such as ventricular compliance (or left ventricular stiffness) and the stroke volume/preload curve is as much influenced by afterload (or resistance in the arterial system) as it is by left ventricular contractility. Occasionally it occurs that cardiac output is maintained at certain preload as long as afterload remains low but becomes inadequate if afterload rises. This, for instance, may be the case after surgical repair of mitral insufficiency in a patient with poor left ventricular function if the leaking mitral valve has provided a low-resistance outflow of blood from the left ventricle and therefore a low afterload. For such situations in which increase of afterload causes a critical change of the stroke-volume/preload curve and consequently ventricular failure, the term "afterload mismatch" has been coined.
Although end-diastolic pressure and stroke volume do not adequately define left ventricular pump function they may be used to monitor changes in the hemodynamic situation. As such changes are relatively easy to assess these parameters can be used for postoperative monitoring.

2.3.2. Parameters derived from the isovolumetric phase of ventricular contraction

The first derivative of the left ventricular pressure curve (dP/dt) is relatively easy to obtain. Its peak value (the steepest rise of ventricular pressure - peak dP/dt), if adequately measured, is a fair measure of left ventricular pump function. Peak dP/dt is not entirely independent of preload and afterload but sufficiently so to be of practical value. Problems are the wide range of normal values (1100 to 2300 mmHg/s) and the lack of isovolumetric contraction in patients with mitral regurgitation.
A more complex parameter is 'V' max which is derived from dP/dt/28P. 'V' max is subject to the same limitations as is peak dP/dt.

2.3.3. Ejection fraction

Ejection fraction (E.F.) is the proportion of the left ventricular volume that is ejected during systole. The following equation is used:

E.F. = (End-diastolic volume - end-systolic volume)/end-diastolic volume.

Calculations of ventricular volumes are usually based upon

the left ventricular angiogram. Ideally, volumes and E.F. are calculated by using two projections of the left ventricle but often only the right anterior oblique projection is used with acceptable results.
Ejection fraction is a suitable parameter to identify patients with very poor left ventricular function but does not allow precise assessment of left ventricular pump function.

2.3.4. The pressure-volume relationship
The relationship between end-systolic volume and end-systolic pressure is one of the best indices currently available to assess left ventricular pump function (3). If the relation is determined under varying circumstances by administration of drugs such as nitroprusside and dobutamine, a line can be constructed that connects the end-systolic pressure - end-systolic volume points and E max and other parameters can be calculated.
Obviously this sophisticated method is rather cumbersome and currently hardly suitable for routine clinical application.

2.3.5. Regional wall motion
The methods described above are all designed to assess total left ventricular pump function. A different approach consists of determining movements of portions of the left ventricular wall separately. Various methods have been proposed to divide the left ventricular contour into separate segments and to express their movements. However, all methods use the same principle and no method has been shown to be clearly superior to the others.
Undoubtedly analysis of regional wall motion is the only method to identify regional differences in contraction pattern and to relate coronary obstructions to changes in the areas they supply. On the other hand it is impossible to reduce the data obtained to a single figure which makes comparison of individual patients very difficult. The method has also limited value in assessing ventricular pump function. Therefore, regional wall motion analysis should be considered in conjunction with other parameters.

Probably our most important conclusion should be that intelligent interpretation of angiographic data requires a good understanding of how they are obtained and what the relative merits and limitations of various parameters are. If used in such a manner and correctly interpreted within the context of the entire clinical picture catheterization data can be tremendously valuable in the selection and management of surgical candidates.

REFERENCES

1. Proudfit WL, Bruschke AVG, MacMillan JP, Williams G.W., Sones F.M. Jr: Fifteen year survival study of patients with obstructive coronary artery disease. Circulation 68:986-997,1983.
2. Baan J, vander Velde ET, de Bruin HG, Smeenk GJ, Koops J,

van Dijk AD, Temmerman D, Senden J, Buis B: Continuous measurement of left ventricular volume in animals and humans by conductance catheter. Circulation 70:812-823,1984.

3. Sagawa K: Editorial: The end-systolic pressure-volume relation of the ventricle: definition, modifications and clinical use. Circulation 63:1223-1227,1981.

TRANSESOPHAGEAL 2-D ECHOCARDIOGRAPHY: A NEW DIMENSION IN CLINICAL CARE

Norbert P. de Bruijn, M.D., Fiona M. Clements, M.D.

Within a decade, echocardiography has become an accepted method for assessing global left ventricular (LV) function, regional myocardial function and morphologic abnormalities. Drawbacks of the standard transthoracic approach are poor image quality in patients with a difficult chest configuration, particularly in those with obesity, emphysema and chronic obstructive pulmonary disease. Application of an ultrasonic transducer is also limited to clinical elective or semi-elective situations in patients who are unencumbered by bandages or monitoring equipment and who can be moved around for imaging. The recent development (1,2) of a miniature ultrasonic phased array transducer for transesophageal imaging of the heart offers a promising means of relatively non invasive assessment of global and regional myocardial function and of morphological abnormalities. Images obtained from the transesophageal approach are generally of high quality when compared to those obtained through the anterior chest wall.

The ultrasonic probe consists of 32 linearly arranged elements with a center frequency of 3.5 MHz. The transducer which measures 14 x 15 x 32 mm is mounted on the tip of a commercially available gastroscope from which the optical fibers have been removed. A 90° sector for real time imaging is obtained by appropriate phasing of the single elements. The images are produced at a frequency of 25 s^{-1}.

At present approximately 20 units are in operation for intraoperative use both for cardiac surgical and general surgical procedures and we estimate that about a thousand patients have been monitored in this way; not a single complication has been described. There are a number of potential complications: the possibility of esophageal abrasions and even perforation has to be kept in mind, as with any device introduced into the esophagus. It is self evident that esophageal pathology, such as strictures, varices, etc. are an absolute contraindication for the insertion of this device. Relative contraindications are gastric reflux, and surgery in the sitting position, where vocal cord paralysis may result from pressure between the endotracheal tube and the ultrasound probe.

The only commercially available unit for transesophageal-2-D echocardiography is produced by Diasonics, but a number of other manufacturers of ultrasound equipment are considering the production of this device as well.

In our practice we introduce the ultrasonic probe immediately after anesthetic induction and endotracheal intubation. The tip of the echoscope is lubricated with a lubricating gel and blindly introduced into the esophagus. In patients who have teeth, both upper and lower teeth are covered by a tooth protector, both to protect them from being damaged and to protect the echoscope.

The ultrasound transducer is then advanced 40-45 cm into the stomach and subsequently is gradually withdrawn until an image of the LV is obtained through the short axis. The plane that we most commonly use for monitoring is a short axis view at the mitral valve level. This view provides both a good assessment of global LV function and enables us to detect regional wall motion abnormalities. (fig.1) (fig.2)

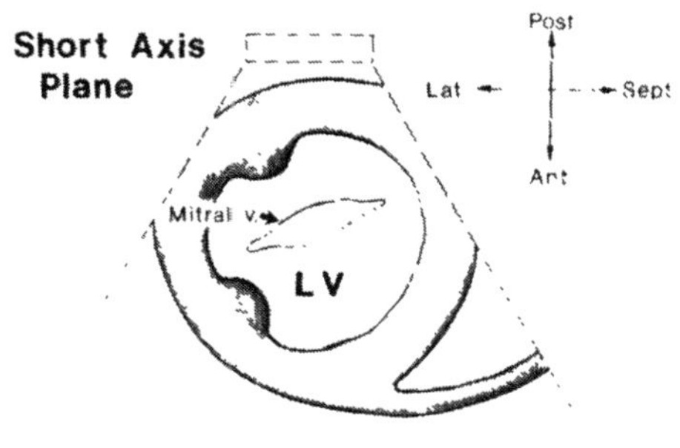

FIGURE 1: Schematic of cross-sectional view on the mitral valve level

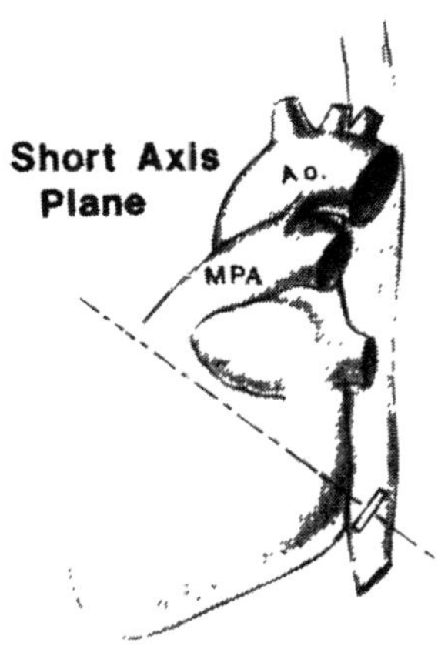

FIGURE 2: Plane of section of short axis view through left and right ventricle

Further withdrawal of the echoscope and angulation of the transducer downwards gives a long axis view of both LV and RV enabling the observer to assess mitral and tricuspid valvular motion as well as measurement (off line) of the long axis diameter of the LV, necessary to calculate a biplane ejection fraction. (fig.3) (fig.4)

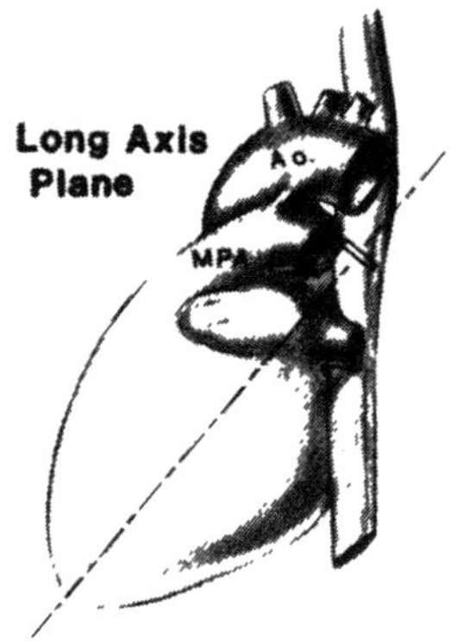

FIGURE 3: Plane of section for LV long axis view or 4 chamber view

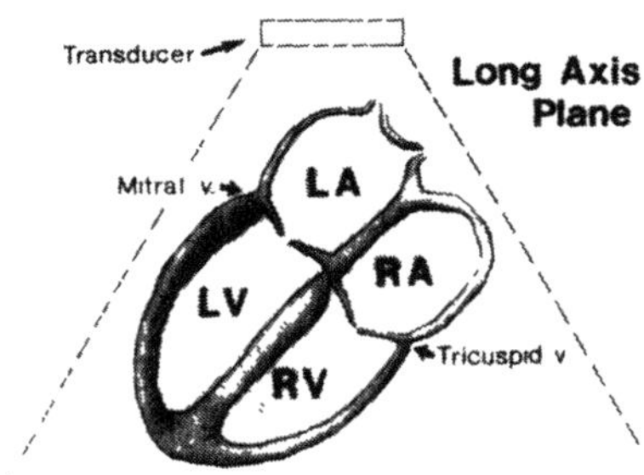

FIGURE 4: Four chamber view

Global LV Function

Apart from on line qualitative assessment of LV function, (3,4) by judging ventricular volume and estimating "contractility", formal analysis of LV pump function is possible only off line. Numerous experimental and clinical studies have documented the reliability of 2-dimensional echocardiography for the quantitation of LV volumes. The biplane area-length method is frequently used and has been shown to be accurate for the determination of LV volumes and ejection fraction (EF). Echocardiography tends to underestimate both end-diastolic and end-systolic volumes to the same degree, so ejection fraction tends to correlate well with cineangiographic data. We studied seven patients undergoing CABG in whom 4 ejection fractions were calculated in the period before cardiopulmonary bypass. TEE images of the LV short axis at the mitral valve level and of the LV long axis were obtained immediately after induction of anesthesia, 5 minutes after skin incision, 5 minutes following median sternotomy and immediately prior to institution of CPB. Using the Franklin Quantic 1200 computer, one beat during each episode was selected and the endocardial outline during end-systole and end-diastole was traced using a bit pad digitizer. The computer subsequently calculated short axis area and major axis length at end-systole and end-diastole and computed ventricular volumes and EF from these data. The mean value of these four determinations was correlated with the preoperative cineangiographic value.

We found a good correlation (R=0.73) between the two methods.(fig.5).

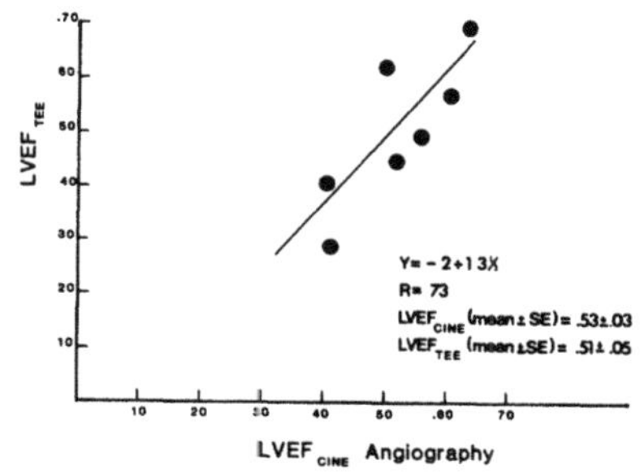

FIGURE 5: Correlation of LV ejection fraction by TEE and cineangiography

Because the transducer has to be repositioned to obtain both a short axis view and a long axis image, when using biplane methods to calculate ventricular volumes this method is not very practical when using transesophageal 2-D-echocardiography as a monitor. Reduction of the short axis area contributes more to ventricular ejection than shortening of the long axis and one may use fractional short axis area change (FAC) as an estimate of pump function. In seven patients undergoing CABG we correlated biplane EF's obtained by 2-D echo with fractional short axis area change and found a good correlation (R=0.82) (fig. 6).

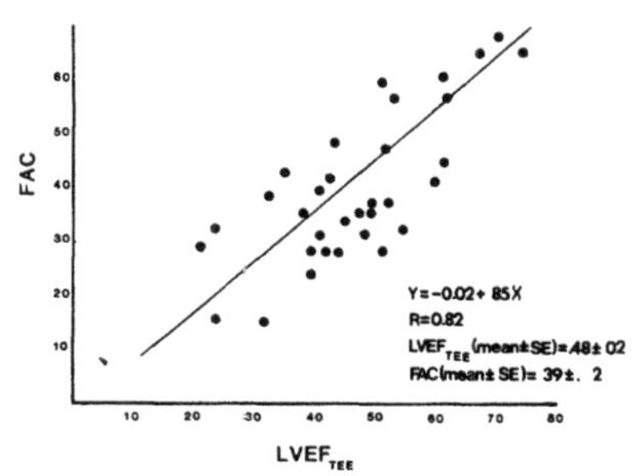

FIGURE 6: Correlation of fractional area change of short axis plane and LV ejection fraction by the biplane method

Whereas the ECG provides some indication of the site of ischemia by virtue of lead placement, hemodynamic parameters allow inference of ischemia only by an effect on global ventricular function. This effect may or may not occur promptly following the onset of ischemia. Furthermore ECG changes of ischemia frequently occur some time after myocardial function has begun to fail, and in the operative setting, lead placement and hence ECG sensitivity may be severely restricted by the sterile surgical field.

It has long been appreciated that an ischemic region of the myocardium fails to contract normally during the cardiac cycle. This has been described by cineangiography and 2-D-echocardiography (s). Such wall motion abnormalities have been described as paradoxical outward movement or failure to move inward during systole and as failure of the myocardium to thicken during systole. For continuous evaluation of WMA a short axis view across the left ventricle at the level of the papillary muscles or the mitral valve has been found to be most useful. For an experienced observer it is very well possible to diagnose existing and new WMA on line in the operating room, and herein lies the real benefit of TEE as a clinical monitor. A more formal analysis of WMA is possible only off line (6). We have used the Franklin Quantic 1200 system to analyze left ventricular wall motion.

In a similar fashion as described above, the endocardial outlines in end-diastole and end-systole are digitized. Subsequently the computer generates, with the aid of an edge-detection program, the endocardial outlines of each frame between end-diastole, end-systole and the second end-diastole. The border is divided into 64 equal segments and WM is then measured with the center line model, which calculates the midpoint between each two frames and then constructs a line perpendicular to the circumference through each midpoint. The length of each of the 64 lines thus generated is a measure for the WM.

Air

When the circulation is restored after CPB, embolization of entrapped intracardiac air represents a significant risk in the patient in whom the left side of the heart has been opened for valve replacement, ablation of abberant pathways, aneurysmectomy, or repairs of congenital malformations. Despite maneuvers developed to expel air from the heart the possibility of air remaining in the left heart chambers is not imaginary and has been responsible for transient or permanent neurologic damage, myocardial infarction and death.

TEE provides an extremely useful tool to detect any residual air, thus alerting the surgical team to repeat maneuvers to remove the air. The problem which has not been solved is to quantitate the amount of air remaining in the heart and determining what amount of air is of clinical relevance.

Shunts

Injection of a bolus of agitated saline, which acts as an echogenic contrast medium can be useful for the detection of intracardiac right-to-left shunts, which will show as contrast appearing in the left heart chambers. Streaming of blood within contrast filled chambers (negative contrast) indicates left-to-right shunting. Injection of contrast into the RV can be helpful in detecting tricuspid insufficiency with regurgitation of contrast into the RA.

Conclusion

Transesophageal-2D-echocardiography is a tool which opens new diagnostic possibilities for the anesthesiologist. Although it has namely been explored in patients undergoing cardiac surgery, perhaps its most exciting application will be in cardiac patients undergoing non-cardiac surgery. The potential of TEE in this type of high risk patients is enormous especially if one considers that it may replace more invasive monitoring like pulmonary artery catheters.

At present cost is still a factor which stands in the way of more general use, but once the transducers will be built in greater quantity and especially once the echocardiographs in present use, which include facilities which are unnecessary in the operating room, have been reduced to the exact needs of the anesthesiologist, the cost will be reduced to a level at which its use would become economically feasible.

New technology is being evaluated at present, providing higher resolution images with smaller size echoscopes. Transesophageal doppler echocardiography allowing the assessment of blood flow rates is being developed and doppler color flow mapping and three-dimensional echocardiography are looming at the horizon.

Finally, the application of this new technology is so easy to learn, that this will form no obstacle for its widespread use in the near future.

References

1. Soquet J, Hanrath L, Zitelli P, et al: Transesophageal phased array for imaging the heart. TEEE 29:707-712, 1982.
2. Schluter M, Langenstein BA, Polster J, et al: Transesophageal cross-sectional echocardiography with a phased array transducer system. Technique and initial clinical results. Br Heart J 48:67-72, 1982.
3. Matsumoto M, Oka Y, Strom J, et al: Application of transesophageal echocardiography to continuous intraoperative monitoring of left ventricular performance. Am J Cardiology 46:95-105, 1980.
4. Matsumoto M, Hanrath P, Kremer P, et al: Evaluation of left ventricular performance during supine exercise by transesophageal M-mode echocardiography in normal subjects. Br Heart J 48:61-66, 1982.
5. Kisslo JA, Robertson D, Gilbert BW, et al: A comparison of real-time, two-dimensional echocardiography and cineangiography in detecting left ventricular asynergy. Circulation 55:134-141, 1977.
6. Moynihan PF, Parisi AF, Feldman CL: Quantitative detection of regional left ventricular contraction abnormalities by two-dimensional echocardiography. 1. Analysis of Methods. Circulation 63:752-760, 1981.

THE EEG AND EVOKED POTENTIALS

J.G. BOVILL

Cardiac surgery with extracorporeal circulation is associated with a series of complex changes, including hypotension, hypothermia and haemodilution. These, together with the effects of anaesthetic and other drugs, can profoundly influence cerebral function. Moderate to high doses of opioids are commonly administered by cardiac anaesthetists. These drugs produce intense miosis, which deprives the anaesthetist of information derived from changes in pupil size. Hypotension is common at the onset of bypass and may result in cerebral ischaemia unless adequately corrected, especially in patients with cerebral vascular disease. Gaseous and particulate matter arising in the extracorporeal system and the effects of haemodilution and non-pulsatile flow may also contribute to brain damage during bypass, despite careful precautions. Monitoring cerebral function is therefore an important responsibility of the cardiac anaesthetist. For this a reliable method of assessing brain activity is needed and traditionally use has been made of the electroencephalogram (EEG).

The EEG, recorded from scalp electrodes, represents the summation of electrical activity generated by postsynaptic potentials from a vast number of neurones, mainly of pyramidal type in the cerebral cortex but also from subcortical nuclei such as the thalamus. These postsynaptic potentials are triggered by chemical transmission across the synapse, which in turn is triggered by the arrival of an axonal depolarization wave (action potential) at the presynaptic membrane. Postsynaptic potentials are of a lower voltage than the action potential and may be either excitatory (depolarizing) or inhibitory (hyperpolarizing). The negative and positive waves recorded in the scalp EEG have been shown to be related to arrival of trains of these inhibitory and excitatory postsynaptic potentials (1). The recorded EEG, however, represents the sampling of potentials from only a very minute fraction, less than 0.3%, of all brain cells.

The processes involved in the generation of postsynaptic potentials utilize considerable energy, derived from oxidative metabolism of glucose in the mitochondriae of neurones. Since brain cells have a very limited reserve of metabolic substrates, anything which prevents delivery of adequate supplies of oxygen and glucose to the brain will be rapidly reflected in EEG changes (2). The EEG is therefore a sensitive monitor of cerebral circulatory insufficiency or hypoxia. There is a high correlation between ipsilateral slowing of the EEG (a characteristic of cerebral ischaemia) and carotid occlusion (3). In the normal healthy individual, changes in the EEG in response to hypoxia do not occur until the oxygen tension of the cerebral venous blood falls below 18 mmHg (2.4 kPa), corresponding to an oxygen saturation of 28%. When this occurs the EEG slows, and amplitude increases. If hypoxia persists intermittent slow waves and periods of flat EEG develop. Eventually the EEG becomes completely flat. Although these changes are initially reversible, with continuing hypoxia and deterioration of the metabolic state of the brain, they finally become irreversible. Deep levels of anaesthesia produce similar EEG patterns and there may be difficulty in distinguishing the EEG signs of hypoxia from those of deepening anaesthesia.

The EEG is a graphic record of waves of electrical potential differences arising between distinct locations on the scalp, with amplitudes varying between 10-200 uV and frequency from 0.5-30 Hz. The rhythmic activity of the EEG is thought to depend, at least partially, on subcortical structures, especially the thalamus (4). The variations in frequency are arbitrarily divided into four groups - alpha rhythm, 7.5-13 Hz; beta rhythm, above 13 Hz; theta rhythm, 3.5-7.5 Hz; delta rhythm, 0.5-3.5 Hz.

The EEG signal is essentially non-periodic - i.e., a pattern does not repeat at fixed intervals - and random. The absence of a regularly recurring pattern in the waveform makes the interpretation of the EEG considerably more complicated than e.g., the ECG. Considerable training and expertise is needed to recognise the characteristic waves and patterns associated with various clinical conditions. Few anaesthetists have either this expertise or the time to apply it, which is one of the reasons why the EEG has attracted less attention than other forms of monitoring. In two recent textbooks on cardiac anaesthesia, fewer than three paragraphs were devoted to electroencephalography. An additional disadvantage of conventional EEG recording in the operating theatre has been the amount of paper generated using conventional registration methods. The commonly used recording speed, 30 mm/sec is the equivalent of 108 metres paper each hour.

Thus in order to make the EEG an attractive and worthwhile form of monitoring for the anaesthetist some form of data reduction is required. A variety of automatic EEG processing techniques have been developed. The first commercially available apparatus that attempted this was the cerebral function monitor (CFM)(5). The CFM monitors the signal from a single EEG derivation, which is filtered between 2-15 Hz and then subjected to further asymmetric filtering which compensates for the inherent tendency of slow waves to have a higher amplitude than faster ones. Rectification produces an average peak amplitude signal, said to be proportional to 'cerebral function', that is written on a strip recorder that can be run at a slow speed (30 cm/hour) for trend analysis. The CFM, originally designed for use in the intensive care unit, has been used as a monitor of cerebral function during cardiopulmonary bypass (6). While CFM recordings can show dramatic changes during periods of global cerebral ischaemia it is less valuable in detection of focal ischaemia. Among the disadvantages of the CFM are its lack of information about frequency and the inability to monitor bilaterally. The successor of the CFM, the cerebral function analysing monitor (CFAM) overcomes most of these problems (8).

The recent advances in computer technology have revolutionised EEG processing, allowing sophisticated analysis to be performed and displayed in real-time. Two main divisions of EEG processing have been described- analysis in the time domain and spectral analysis in the frequency domain. Analysis in the time domain is primarily concerned with the variation in signal amplitude with time but, by use of techniques such as period analysis to measure the wavelengths between baseline crossings (zero crossings) of the EEG, indirect information about the frequency composition of the signal can be obtained. This technique is analogous to the way which the human observer estimates the frequency content of an epoch of EEG recording. Various techniques of period and period-amplitude analysis have been described, including the Klein analyzer (9) and the CFAM mentioned earlier. The Neurometrics Monitor[R] uses aperiodic analysis (10) to present each wave form in relationship to its frequency, amplitude and time of occurrence in a concentrated format on a colour video-monitor. The use of frequency data derived from zero-corssing methods as a measure of EEG activity has been criticised (11) since the frequency histograms generated are not uniquely related to that EEG and several different waveforms can generate the same zero-cross frequencies. This problem can be overcome by applying zero-crossing analysis not only to the original signal but also to the first and second derivatives of the signal. In cardiac surgery periodic-amplitude analysis has been found to be effective both on grounds of safety and cost (12).

Analysis in the frequency domain involves transformation of the amplitude-time relationship of the EEG to give the relationship between frequency and amplitude, or more often, power. The use of power, which is amplitude squared, reflects the origins of this form of analysis in engineering science. The most commonly used technique is the Fast Fourier Transformation (FFT), which decomposes the signal into sine waves of differing amplitude although others can be used. The use of the Walsh transformation, based on orthogonal rectangular functions, rather than sinusoidal functions, to generated EEG spectra has been described (13); this gives the same information as the FFT but is attractive because it requres less computer time. Frequency transformations are applied to successive intervals, or epochs, of the EEG and the resulting power spectrums smoothed and then displayed on a monitoring device such as a CRT or paper recorder (Fig. 1). Epochs can vary from 2 sec to several minutes but it must be realised that additional time, up to 50% of the epoch duration, will be needed for the necessary computations and display. Thus spectral analysis techniques are unsuitable for detection of events with a short duration e.g. spikes or the presence of burst suppression during anaesthesia.

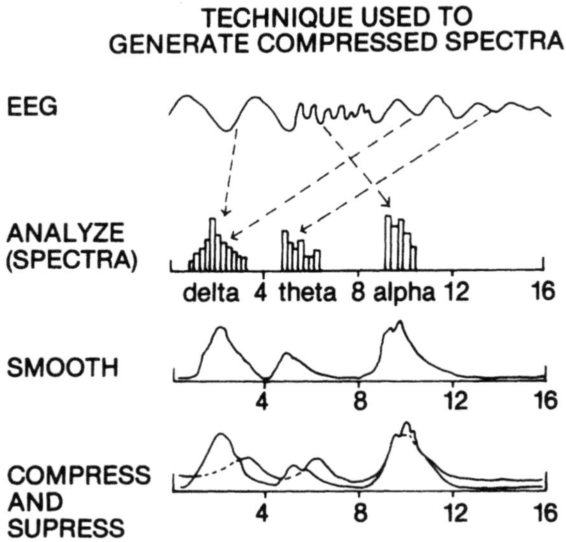

Figure 1. Generation of Compressed Spectral Array (CSA).

A variety of methods are available for the display of power spectra. The first, and still most widely used, is the compressed spectral array (CSA) developed by Bickford (14). In the CSA the spectrum of each epoch is plotted as a graph of power versus frequency. By shifting the origin vertically for each succeeding epoch and applying hidden-line suppression techniques, the familiar patterns of "hills and valleys" is displayed (Fig. 2). The CSA has been used to evaluate EEG changes produced by hypotension during cardiopulmonary bypass (15) and to evaluate anaesthetic depth (16). Despite the attractiveness of the CSA display it is not ideal. The use of hidden-line suppression tends to obscure information, especially when high-amplitude activity is present, so that subsequent low-amplitude activity at the same frequency in following epochs is hidden from view. This problem has been overcome by the technique of "Density Modulation" (17) in which the spectrum is displayed not as a graph but as a line of varying density or a series of dots of various sizes. Areas of maximum intensity then correspond to those frequencies making the largest contribution to the spectrum. This allows changes in the EEG to be earlier and easier seen than with the CSA display.

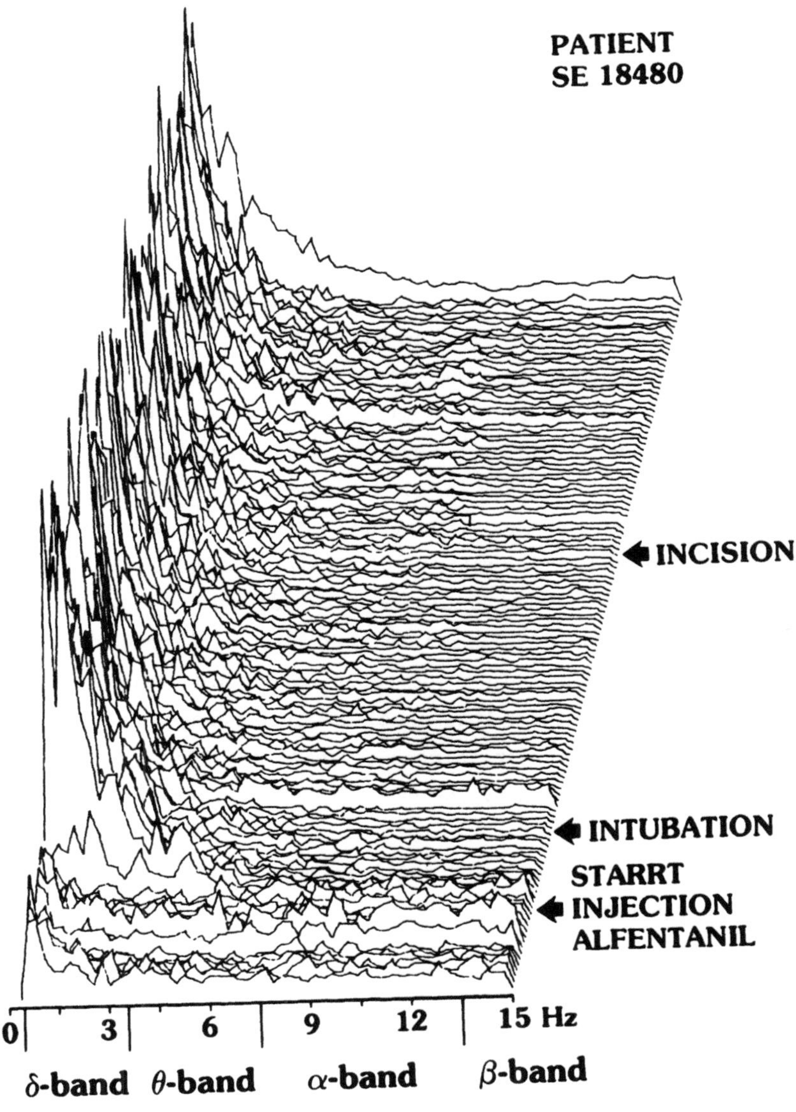

Figure 2. Example of CSA showing changes produced by induction of anaesthesia with alfentanil 125 ug/kg.

What benefits does routine EEG monitoring offer the cardiac anaesthetist and the patient? The most important role of EEG monitoring is the timely detection of reversible changes in cerebral function. This is of most value during cardiopulmonary bypass, especially in patients with occlusive cerebrovascular disease. EEG abnormalities are common at the onset of bypass and appear to be related to the concurrent decrease in mean blood pressure. In most patients these changes have a shorter duration than the period of hypotension, presumably due to autoregulation of cerebral blood flow, which is negligibly affected by hypothermia above 20° C (18). Attempts have been made to define lower safe limits of perfusion pressure. Prior (19) found a higher threshold (36 $\pm$ 9 mmHg) for EEG abnormalities in older and hypertensive patients than in younger normotensive patients (27 $\pm$ 10 mmHg). However anaesthetists deal with individuals, not groups, and without the aid of EEG monitoring it is impossible to determine the optimal perfusion pressure for our patients. For patients with cerebrovascular disease, decreases in perfusion pressure of as little as 5 mmHg below the individuals critical value may result in significant cerebral ischaemia. Although hypothermia causes significant EEG changes (20), these are readily distinguished from these due to cerebral ischaemia. Patients with chronic cerebral ischaemia, particularly following a stroke, may not demonstrate EEG abnormalities, even when marginal perfusion is present, unless recordings from several derivations are made. In these patients, consideration should be given to use of conventional multichannel EEG recordings done by an experienced electroencephalographer, since most commercially available EEG analysing apparatuses provide only for dual channel recordings.

The EEG may also be of value in predicting neurological outcome when EEG abnormalities persist. Schwarz et al (21), using the CFM, had a 83% success rate in predicting either uncomplicated recovery or neurological deficit in 100 patients.

Evoked Potentials

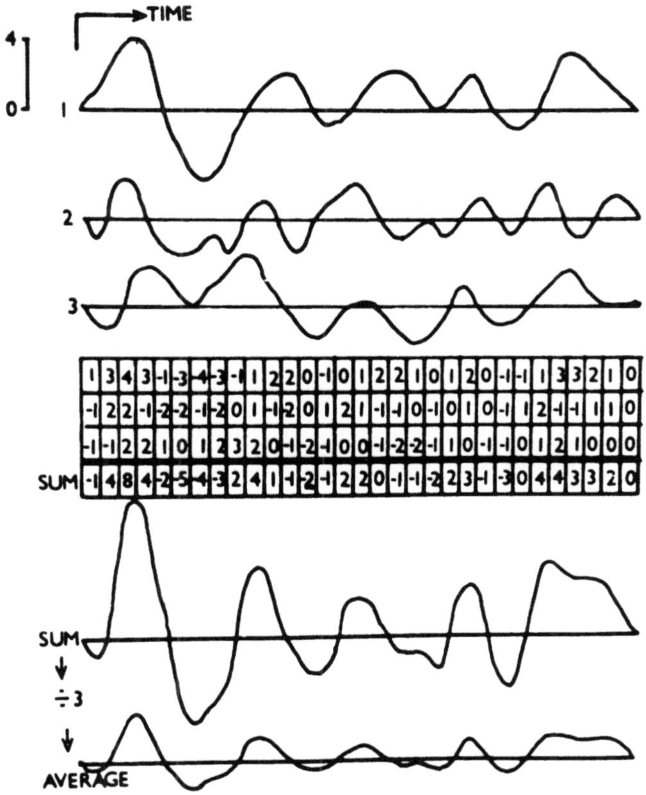

Figure 3. Principle of averaging for acquisition of sensory evoked potentials.

Sensory evoked potentials (SEP) are electrical responses generated within the nervous system in response to sensory stimulation. The evoking stimulus may be either visual, auditory or somatosensory. Visual stimuli may be either a light flash or a changing pattern on a television screen (pattern reversal). For auditory evoked responses, a series of sounds, either clicks or tone bursts, are presented via headphones. The most common form of somatosensory stimulus is a constant current electrical potential applied over a peripheral nerve, e.g. median nerve at the wrist or posterior tibial nerve at the ankle. Other stimuli are occassionally used such as finger tapping, vibration or heat. SEPs have a low amplitude (1-5 uV) compared to that of the background EEG (10-200 uV) so that it is usually impossible to extract the evoked potential from a single stimulus. Fortunately the evoked potential always occurs a fixed interval after the applied stimulus i.e. it is time-locked to the stimulus. Thus by using computerised averaging and giving repeated stimuli it is possible to extract the SEP. The principle of averaging is illustrated in Fig. 3. The number of stimulus repetitions needed to achieve a satisfactory response (good signal to noise ratio) depends on the amplitude of the single evoked potential and varies from 50-60 for visual evoked responses to 2000 or more for brain-stem evoked potentials.

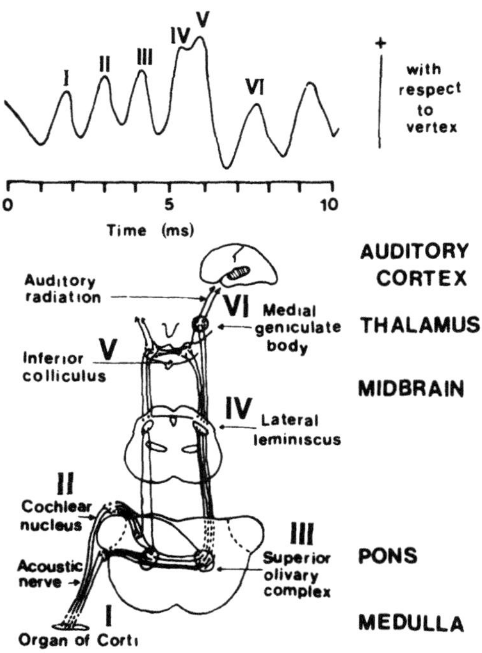

Figure 4. Brain-stem auditory evoked potential waveform showing origins of the labelled peaks.

Considerably more repetitions are required to obtain a "clean" response if there is much interference in the input signal to the averager e.g., from muscle activity, ECG or extraneous electrical interference. The improvement in the signal to noise ratio is proportional to N^2 (N = no. of repetitions).

SEPs reflect the functional integrity of specific sensory pathways. This can be best illustrated by the brain-stem auditory evoked potential (BAEP) where individual peaks in the waveform are known to arise from well defined structures in the auditory pathways (Fig. 4). SEPs are valuable diagnostic tools in neurology, audiology and ophthalmology. They are also increasingly used in neurosurgery, especially during posterior fossa surgery and surgery in the region of the optic nerve and chiasma.

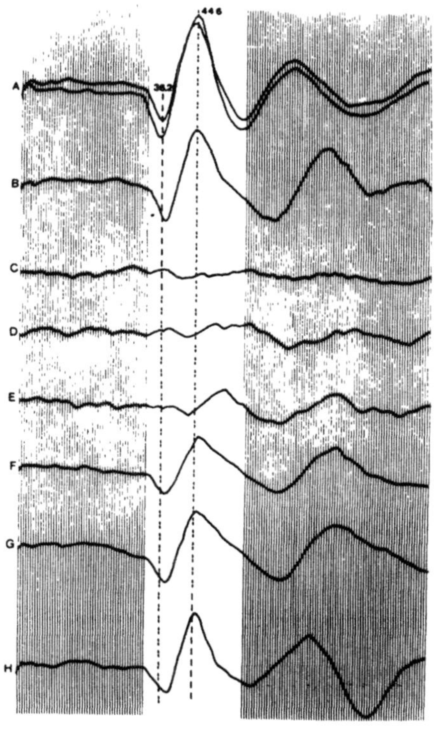

Figure 5. Posterior tibial nerve SSEP during aortic surgery. A is the recording made before anaesthesia and B the postinduction recording. At C the waveform dissappeared with clamping the aorta, returning when the clamp was removed at E.

Somatosensory evoked potentials (SSEP) are valuable in monitoring spinal cord function during scoliosis surgery. Although the usefulness of SEP monitoring has not been evaluated in cardiac surgery, SSEPs have proven of value in aortic surgery e.g. removal of aortic aneurysms and repair of coarctations, when there is a risk of spinal cord ischaemia during periods of aortic clamping. In these situations early warning of a deterioration in cord function, reflected by a loss of the SSEP (Fig. 5) can allow speedy corrective measures to be taken and thereby prevent the occurrence of disastrous paraplegia.

REFERENCES

1. Schmidt RF: Fundamentals of Neurophysiology. New York: Springer Verlag, 1978.
2. Ingvar DH, Sjoelund B, Ardoe A: Correlation between dominant EEG frequency, cerebral oxygen uptake and blood flow. Electroenceph Clin Neurophysiol 41:268-276, 1976.
3. Sundt TM, Houser OW, Sharbrough FW, et al: Carotid endarterectomy: Results, complications and monitoring techniques. Advances in Neurology, Vol 16, Edited by Thompson RA, Green Jr. New York, Raven Press, pp 97-119, 1977.
4. Niedermeyer E, Lopas da Silva FH: Electroencephalography: Basic principles, clinical applications and related fields. Urban and Schwarzberg, Munich, 1982.
5. Maynard DE, Prior PF, Scott DF: Device for continuous monitoring of cerebral activity in resuscitated patients. Br Med J 4:545-546, 1969.
6. Branthwaite MA: Prevention of neurological damage during open-heart surgery. Thorax 30:258-261, 1975.
7. Cucchiara RF, Sharbrough FW, Messick JM, et al: An electroencephalographic filter-processor as an indicator of cerebral ischemia during carotid endarterectomy. Anesthesiology 51:77-79, 1979.
8. Maynard DE: Development of the CFM: The cerebral function analysing monitor. Ann Anesth Franç 20:253-255, 1979.
9. Klein FF: A waveform analyzer applied to the human EEG. IEEE Trans Biomed Eng BME 23:246-252, 1976.

10. Demetrescu M: The aperiodic character of the electroencephalogram: A new approach to data analysis and condensation. Physiologist 18:189, 1975.
11. Levy WJ, Shapiro HM, Maruchak G, Meathe E: Automated EEG processing for intraoperative monitoring. A comparison of techniques. Anesthesiology 53:223-236, 1980.
12. Pronk RAF: EEG processing in Cardiac Surgery. Report R-1982-1. Utrecht: Instituut Medical Physics TNO, 1982.
13. Dzwonczyk R, Howie MB, McDonald JS, Lingam RP: Walsh versus fourier analysis of the electroencephalogram (EEG) during anesthesia. Anesthesiology 59:A171, 1983.
14. Bickford RG, Billinger TW, Flemming NI, et al: The compressed spectral array (CSA) - a pictorial EEG. Proc San Diege Biomed Symp 11:365-370, 1972.
15. Stockard JJ, Bickford RG, Schauble JF: Pressure-dependent cerebral ischaemia during cardiopulmonary bypass. Neurology 23:521-529, 1973.
16. Berezowskyj JL, McEwan JA, Anderson GB, et al: A study of anaesthesia depth by power spectral analysis of the electroencephalogram. Can Anaesth Soc J 23:1-8, 1976.
17. Fleming RA, Smith NT: Density modulation: A technique for the display of three-variable data in patient monitoring. Anesthesiology 50: 543-546, 1979.
18. Fox LS, Blackstone EH, Kirklin JW, et al: Relationship of whole body oxygen consumption to perfusion flow rate during hypothermic cardiopulmonary bypass. J Thoracic Cardiovasc Surg 83:239-248, 1982.
19. Prior PF: EEG monitoring and evoked potentials in brain ischaemia. Br J Anaesth 57:63-81, 1985.
20. Levy WJ: Quantitative analysis of EEG changes during hypothermia. Anesthesiology 60:291-297, 1984.
21. Schwartz MS, Colvin MP, Prior PF, et al: The cerebral function monitor: its value in predicting the neurological outcome in patients undergoing cardiopulmonary bypass. Anaesthesia 28:611-618, 1973.

PREOPERATIVE MEDICATION: MAINTENANCE OR MODIFICATION

P.J. HENNIS

The anesthesiologist visiting patients scheduled for cardiac surgery may be confronted with a list of drugs for the heart that is both long and impressive. Does he maintain or modify all these drugs? I will try to answer this question, first, by narrowing the subject to adult patients with coronary artery disease and/or valve lesions, since they form the majority of patients undergoing cardiac surgery. Second, by understanding "maintenance" as continuation of the same dosage regimen of a drug and "modification" as changing drug dosage or discontinuation of the drug(s).

What drugs do we talk about? To illustrate the incidence of preoperative medication, I reviewed 320 adult patients, who were scheduled to undergo coronary artery bypass grafting (CABG) surgery and/or valvular replacement, during the second half year of 1984 in the University Hospital of Leiden. Of these 320 patients, 196 were scheduled for CABG surgery, 84 for valvular replacement, and 40 for both types of surgery. The CABG patients mostly took a combination of a beta-blocking drug, a calcium antagonist and a nitrate (fig. 1).

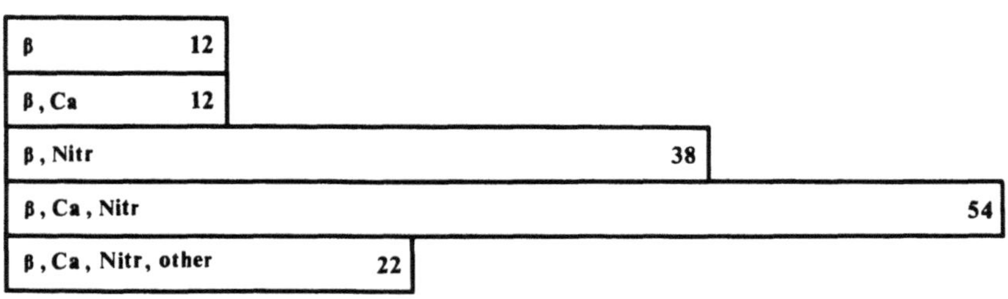

Fig. 1: Preoperative medication for patients scheduled for CABG surgery In most patients (138 of 191), medication consisted of a beta-blocking drug (β) alone, or together with a calcium antagonist (Ca) and a nitrate (Nitr). Other drugs included diuretics, antiarrhythmic agents or vasodilating drugs.

Patients scheduled for valvular replacement mostly took digoxin plus a diuretic (fig. 2).

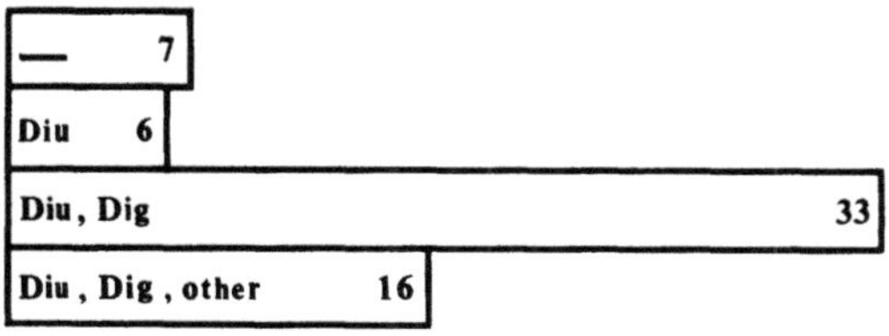

Fig. 2: Preoperative medication for patients scheduled for valvular replacement during the second half year of 1984 in the University Hospital of Leiden. Most patients (55 of 84) took a diuretic (Diu) and/or digoxin (Dig). 7 Patients had no medication. Other drugs included nitrates, anti–arrhythmic and inotropic drugs.

Thus, beta–blocking drugs, calcium antagonists, nitrates, digoxin and diuretics are the drugs that we deal with most often. I believe this drug armamentarium is representative for most centres.

1. **Beta–blocking drugs**

Since the introduction of propranolol, many beta–blocking drugs have been introduced (fig. 3).

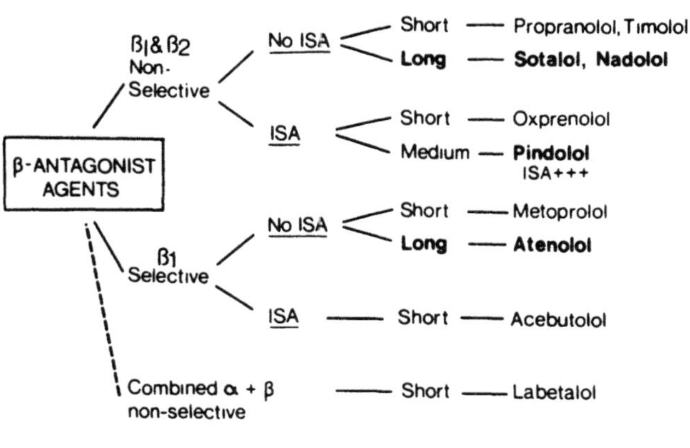

Fig. 3: Classification of some beta–blocking drugs. ISA: intrinsic sympathomimetic activity. [From Opie LH: Drugs and the Heart. I. Beta–blocking agents. Lancet 1:693–698,1980. Reproduced with permission of the author]

All antagonize the actions of catecholamines on beta–adrenoreceptors by competitive inhibition. Some like metroprolol and atenolol are more potent at β_1 than at β_2 receptors, i.e., are said to be more cardio-selective. This cardioselective action is however dose–dependent, i.e., at higher dosage, these drugs become non–selective like propranolol.[1] Apart from effects on β_1 and β_2 receptors, some beta–blocking drugs may have intrinsic sympathomimetic activity (ISA), supplying a basic sympathetic tone (higher resting heart rate) and being less cardiodepressive, like pindolol.[2] Despite the vast choice of agents, all beta–blocking drugs are effective as anti–anginal drugs.[1] Apart from anti–anginal effects, beta–blocking drugs may be used in the treatment of hypertension; both indications are often met in coronary artery disease patients. In addition they may be used as anti–arrythmic drugs, which indication is less frequently met for these patients. All beta–blocking drugs decrease oxygen demand by

1. reducing the increase in heart rate in response to exercise
2. reducing myocardial contractility;

Both processes demand oxygen. By decreasing heart rate, coronary artery perfusion time during diastole will be longer and thus, oxygen supply may be increased.

When are beta–blocking drugs effective? Beta–blocking drugs are effective when patients respond to exercise with an increase in heart rate to less than 100 bpm, while heart rate at rest is approximately 50–60 bpm. In the clinical situation, this is the response of beta–blocking drugs that is usually measured and on what basis dosage regimen is instituted. A second method of response measurement is reduction of isoproterenol–induced tachycardia.[3] However, this may be dangerous (tachycardia, arrhythmias) and appears to be unpleasant. During surgery, a heart rate of 80 or less may be the aim.

Variability in plasma concentrations and thus, response for a certain dose is large[4–6] (fig. 4) and is largely dependent on

1. absorption kinetics; individual variability in absorption from the gut may lead to pharmaceutical availabilities that vary

between 20—70%;

2. Variability in first pass effects, i.e., uptake by the liver, may lead to bioavailabilities of 10—40%.

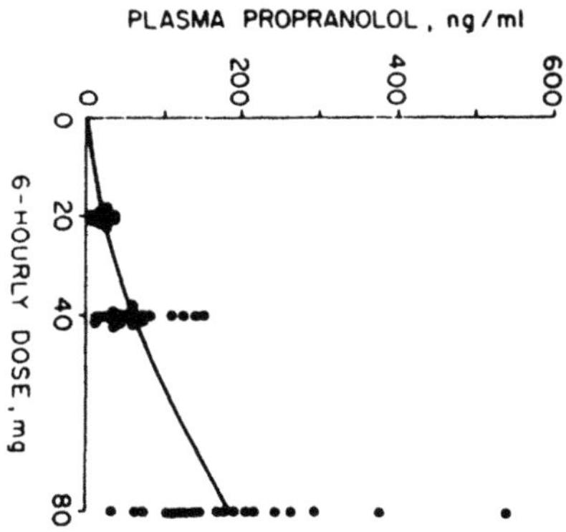

Fig. 4: Plasma concentrations of propranolol during various oral doses. Each dot represents the concentration in one patient. Note the wide range of concentrations at a given dose. [From: Nies AS and Shand DG: Circulation 52:6—15,1975. Reproduced with permission of the author]

For example, the presence of food in the stomach influences the bioavailability and thus plasma concentrations for beta—blocking drugs. For propranolol and metoprolol, two lipophylic drugs, plasma concentrations are higher when these drugs are ingested together with food than when they are ingested without food (on an empty stomach)[7] (fig. 5). The opposite is true for the more hydrophylic drug atenolol.[8] Thus, a patient scheduled for surgery, taking metoprolol on the morning of surgery on an empty stomach will have lower plasma concentrations than in a normal situation, resulting in less reduction of excercise— or stress—induced tachycardia. In contrast, a patient taking atenolol on the morning of surgery may have higher plasma concentrations and more reduction of exercise—induced tachycardia.

What is the relation between plasma concentration and effect for beta—blocking drugs, i.e., their pharmacodynamics? Mullane et al. studied volunteers between 20 and 40 years old, who ingested propranolol 80—160 mg/day, divided over 1—4 doses.[9] Just before the 8 o'clock morning dose, plasma concentrations were 5 to 15 ng/ml with a reduction in excercise heart rate from —10 to —20 bpm. This plasma concentration and reduction of tachycardia was only dependent on dose and <u>not</u> on dose frequency. Significant beta—blockade started with plasma concentrations of 0.5 ng/ml and increased rapidly between concentrations of 0.5 and 20 ng/ml. Above

80 ng/ml, beta-blockade did not increase further.

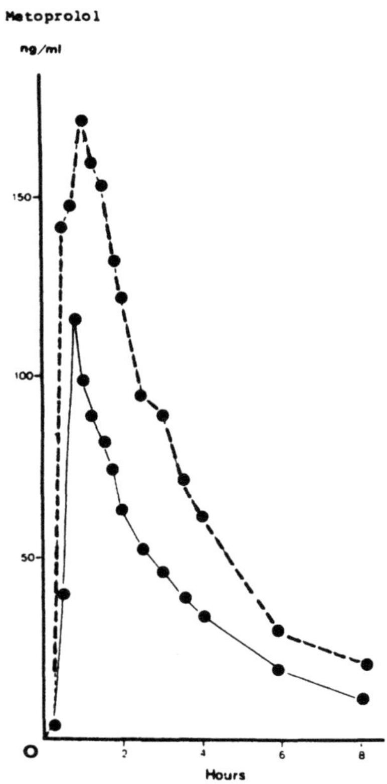

Fig. 5: Plasma concentrations of metoprolol in two healthy volunteers after ingestion of 100 mg metoprolol on an empty stomach (solid line) and together with a standardized breakfast (broken line). [From: Melander A, et al: Clin Pharmacol Ther 22:108-112, 1977. Reproduced with permission of the author]

In a clinical study, measuring percent change in heart rate in response to stress, Sill et al in 1984, found that between concentrations of 0-90 ng/ml, there was a significant correlation between log propranolol plasma concentration and the magnitude of hemodynamic responses (heart rate, blood pressure) to intubation and surgical stimulation.[10] However, in several patients, plasma concentrations were not different from zero (fig. 6). Thus, after oral therapy alone and not administering the morning dose, plasma concentrations may be too low during intubation and surgical stimulation to prevent an increase in heart rate. Probably it can be advocated that beta-blocking therapy is maintained up to the morning of surgery and even be expanded to the prebypass period. For example, if heart rate in response to insertion of cannulas is 100-120, a beta-blocking drug, e.g., pindolol or propranolol is titrated intravenously to reduce this stimulus-induced tachycardia. Thus, beta-blocking therapy is not just stopped when the patients arrives in the operation theatre.

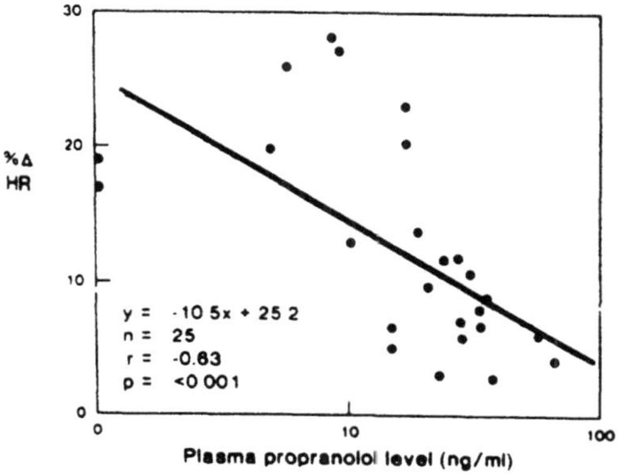

Fig. 6: Correlation of % heart rate change from prelaryngoscopy to postintubation versus the log plasma propranolol concentration. [From: Sill JC et al, Anesthesiology 60:455-463, 1984. Reproduced with permission of the author]

Apart from the above mentioned, there are other reasons to maintain beta-blocking drugs. First, not related to anesthesia, mortality and reinfarctions are reduced in patients who survived acute myocardial infarction as has been demonstrated for timolol and alprenolol.[11,12] Second, related to anesthesia, continuation of beta-blocking therapy, with whatever blocker, has no untoward hemodynamic effects during surgery under various anesthetic regimes.[13-16] Third, acute withdrawal of beta-blocking drugs may precipitate myocardial ischemia and even infarction before surgery starts.[17] Fourth, continuation may be beneficial, since hypertensive crises and dysrhythmia's are less frequent per- and postoperatively.[15] It is interesting to realize that most authors state that it is not dangerous to maintain beta-blocking drugs rather than saying it is beneficial. Thus, one could simply say: regardless of dose, dosage interval and beta-blocking drugs used, do not withdraw (modify), but **maintain.**

2. Calcium antagonists

In contrast to beta-blocking drugs, which share similar effects, calcium-antagonists differ in their effects (fig. 7). Verapamil has a more pronounced effect on electrical conduction in the heart, while nifedipine is more effective in reducing peripheral resistance by arteriolar dilation.[18,19] For both drugs, reflex sympathetic activity may increase

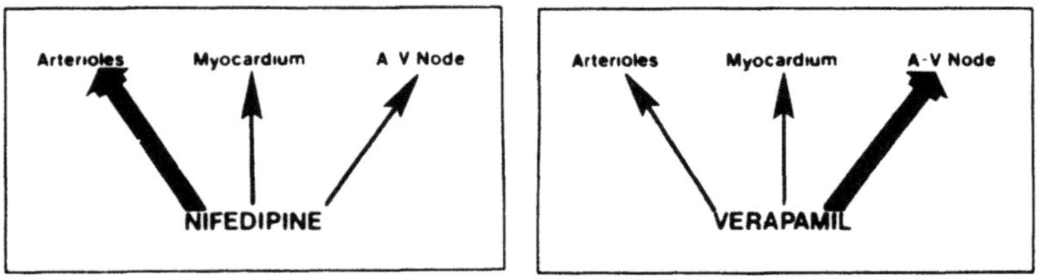

Fig. 7: Cardiovascular effects of nifedipine and verapamil. [From: Reves JG et al, Anesthesiology 57:504–518, 1982. Reproduced with permission of the author]

heart rate and cardiac output, thus partially counterbalancing their negative inotropic effects. The pharmacokinetics of calcium antagonists are more or less comparable to that of beta–blocking drugs. However, in contrast to beta–blocking drugs, the pharmacodynamics have not been studied extensively. A problem here is: how can we measure response in clinical practice, like heart rate changes for beta–blocking drugs? How can we judge whether a patient is adequately "calcium–antagonized"? Even more difficult, how can we judge on a dose–concentration–response basis whether to maintain or modify the combination of a beta–blocking drug plus a calcium antagonist?

Controlled studies on the hemodynamic consequences of maintenance of calcium antagonists, alone or combined with beta–blocking drugs, are lacking. Most information is based on experimental studies in animals, empirical and dependent on the type of anesthetic agents used.

Since inhalational anesthetics interfere with calcium flux across cell membranes, they may be considered to be calcium antagonists or at least calcium entry blockers.[19] Thus, one might expect addition (or potentiation) of negative inotropic, chronotropic and dromotropic effects when calcium antagonists are maintained and inhalational anesthesia is to be given. Indeed these additive effects of verapamil and halothane, enflurane and isoflurane have been demonstrated in dogs.[20–22] Thus, if halothane anesthesia is to be given to patients scheduled for bypass surgery, one might adjust halothane dosage.[19] In fact, verapamil reduces MAC of halothane by 25% in dogs.[23] For nifedipine and inhalational agents, a similar additive negative inotropic effect was shown, but no dromotropic effect, since nifedipine has less effects on conduction than verapamil.[19] Both, probably additive, effects of the combination may be reversed by calcium with more or less success. However, if a patient is then also receiving a beta-blocking drug, these additive effects may even be more pronounced[24] and may not be that easily reversed by calcium. When verapamil is administered to patients on beta-blocking drugs, a third-degree atrioventricular block or even asystole may develop.[25]

In non-inhalational anesthesia, the combined effects of calcium antagonists and beta-blocking drugs may be less outspoken. In fact, Skarvan recently saw no ontoward effects of maintaining the combination while a balanced anesthetic technique was used.[26] Neither is it our impression that during high dose opioid anesthesia maintenance of calcium antagonists together with beta-blocking drugs is a problem.

3. **Nitrates** are the third cornerstone of anti-anginal therapy and the oldest. Their mechanism of action is mostly due to venodilation more than arteriolar dilation. This venodilation leads to a reduced preload, by which ventricular end-diastolic volume is reduced and therefore wall stress is lowered. Thus oxygen demand is lowered[27,28] (fig. 8).

NITRATES:

venodilation → preload
preload → wall stress
wall stress → oxygen demand

arteriolar dilation
(coronary arteries) → oxygen supply

A second beneficial effect may exist on the oxygen supply side due to dilation of coronary arteries. Preoperatively nitroglycerin may be administered as an ointment with a long duration of effect or in the oral or sublingual form. In general it is advocated to **maintain** these drugs up to the morning of surgery. Ointments can be removed before induction as soon as an i.v. drip of nitroglycerin is started.

4. **Digoxin** has a narrow therapeutic window, i.e. toxicity (conduction block) may easily develop when conditions of the patient change. Moreover, the concomitant administration of calcium antagonists, beta–blocking drugs and various antiarrythmic drugs like quinidine, influence the pharmacokinetics of digoxin, leading to higher plasma concentrations and enhancing toxicity.[29,30] Also, potassium changes and changes in renal clearance may modify (therapeutic window) concentration. In general it is advised: **do not continue,**[31] unless ventricular response in atrial fibrillation, where this drug is first choice, is above 90 bpm the day before operation. To test the adequacy of digitalization preoperatively, one could subject a patient to a short walk and judge heart rate. As for its inotropic action, discontinuation on the day of surgery may be safe, since we have potent and immediately acting inotropic drugs such as dopamine and dobutamine at hand.

5. **Diuretics**: are probably best to be **discontinued** for three reasons. First, when patients are in bed, they tend not to accumulate interstitial fluids. Second, it is safer and probably easier to induce anesthesia in a patient who is not volume depleted. Third, diuretics, if to be continued with digoxin, may induce potassium depletion with risk of digoxin toxicity.[29]

Apparently **most preoperative medication should be continued or maintained**; I tried to list some reasons for doing so. However, much more information is needed to study the effects of simultaneous administration of drugs especially if we want to refine dosage regimen. Only then more defined pros and cons of maintenance or modification can be given. Anesthesia and preopeative medication is not to be read from a cook book. Like H.D. Thoreau said: any fool can make a rule and every fool will mind it.

REFERENCES

1. Kehler CH, Fogdall RP: Inotropic agonists and antagonists. In: Acute Cardiovascular Management. Edited by Ream AK, Fogdall RP. Lippincott, Philadelphia, 1982, pp 318–364

2. Man in 't Veld AJ, Schalekamp MADH: How intrinsic sympathomimetic activity modulates the haemodynamic responses to beta-adrenoreceptor antagonists. A clue to the nature of their antihypertensive mechanism. Br J Clin Pharmacol 13 (Suppl):245-257, 1982
3. Dagnino J, Prys-Roberts C: Assessment of β-adrenoreceptor blockade during anesthesia in humans: use of isoproterenol dose-response curves. Anesth Analg 64:305-311, 1985
4. Johnsson G, Regårdh CG: Clinical Pharmacokinetics of β-adrenoreceptor agents. Clin Pharmacokinet 1:233-263, 1976
5. Nies AS, Shand DG: Clinical pharmacology of propranolol. Circulation 52:6-15, 1975
6. Routledge PA, Shand DG: Clinical pharmacokinetics of propranolol. Clin Pharmacokinet 4:73-90, 1979
7. Melander A, Danielson K, Schersten B, Wåhlin E: Enhancement of the bioavailability of propranolol and metoprolol by food. Clin Pharmacol Ther 22:108-112, 1977.
8. Melander A, Stenberg P, Liedholm H, et al: Food-induced reduction in bioavailability of atenolol. Eur J Clin Pharmacol 16:327-330, 1979
9. Mullane JF, Kaufman J, Dvornik D, et al: Propranolol dosage, plasma concentration, and beta blockade. Clin Pharmacol Ther 32:692-700, 1982
10. Sill JC, Nugent M, Moyer TP, et al: Influence of propranolol plasma levels on hemodynamics during coronary artery bypass surgery. Anesthesiology 60:455-463, 1984
11. The Norwegian Multicenter Study Group: Timolol-induced reduction in mortality and reinfarction in patients surviving acute myocardial infarction. N Engl J Med 304:801-807, 1981
12. Andersen MP, Bechsgaard P, Frederikson J, et al: Effect of alprenolol on mortality among patients with definite or suspected acute myocardial infarction: preliminary results. Lancet 2:865-868, 1979
13. Jones EL, Kaplan JA, Dorney ER, et al: Propranolol therapy in patients undergoing myocardial revascularization. Am J Cardiol 38:696-700, 1976
14. Kopriva CJ, Brown ACD, Pappas G: Hemodynamics during general anesthesia in patients receiving propranolol. Anesthesiology 48:28-33, 1978

15. Oka Y, Frishman W, Becker RM, et al: Clinical Pharmacology of the new beta-adrenergic blocking drugs. Part 10. Beta-adrenoreceptor blockade and coronary artery surgery. Am Heart J 99:255–269, 1980
16. Slogoff S, Keats AS, Ott E: Preoperative propranolol therapy and aortocoronary bypass operation. JAMA 240:1487–1490, 1978
17. Pontén J, Häggendal J, Milocco J, et al: Long-term metoprolol therapy and neurolept anesthesia in coronary artery surgery: withdrawal versus maintenance of β_1-adrenoreceptor blockade. Anesth Analg 62:380–390, 1983
18. Henry PD: Comparative pharmacology of calcium antagonists: nifedipine, verapamil and diltiazem. Am J Cardiol 46:1047–1058, 1980
19. Reves JG, Kissin I, Lell WA, et al: Calcium entry blockers: uses and implications for anesthesiologists. Anesthesiology 57:504–518, 1982
20. Kapur PA, Flacke WE: Epinephrine induced arrhythmias and cardiovascular function after verapamil during halothane anesthesia in the dog. Anesthesiology 55:218–225, 1981
21. Kapur PA, Flacke WE, Olewine SK: Comparison of effects of isoflurane versus enflurane on cardiovascular and catecholamine responses to verapamil in dogs. Anesth Analg 61:193–194, 1982
22. Tosone SR, Reves JG, Kissin J, et al: Nifedipine and halothane: additive hemodynamic depression in dogs. Anesth Analg 61:218–219, 1982
23. Maze M, Mason DM, Kates RE: Verapamil decreases MAC for halothane in dogs. Anesthesiology 59:327–329, 1983
24. Packer MP, Meller J, Medina N, et al: Hemodynamic consequences of combined beta-adrenergic and slow calcium channel blockade in man. Circulation 65:660–668, 1982
25. Benaim ME: asystole after verapamil. Br Med J 2:169–170, 1972
26. Skarvan K: Preoperative nifedipine treatment and anesthesia in patients with coronary heart disease. Anesthesiology 59:362–363, 1983
27. Ammon JR, Fogdall RP: Vasoactive drugs. In: Acute Cardiovascular Management. Edited by Ream AK, Fogdall RP. Lippincott, Philadelphia, 1982, pp 366–372
28. Opie LH, Ihadani U: Nitrates. In: Drugs for the Heart. Edited by Opie LH, Grune & Stratton, 1984, pp 23–37

29. Marcus FI, Opie LH, Sonnenblick EH: Digitalis and sympathomimetic stimulants. In: Drugs for the Heart. Edited by Opie LH, Grune & Stratton, 1984, pp 99–115

30. Belz GG, Doering W, Munkes R, et al: Interaction between digoxin and calcium antagonists and antiarrhythmic drugs. Clin Pharmacol Ther 33:410–417, 1983

31. Garman JK, Fogdall RP: The prebypass period. In: Acute Cardiovascular Management. Edited by Ream AK, Fogdall RP. Lippincott, Philadelphia, 1982, pp 402–404

PREOPERATIVE EVALUATION OF THE PATIENT WITH MITRAL VALVE DISEASE

B. Amari, M. Merli, C. Cattani

In recent years, more and more patients have undergone cardiovascular surgery for coronary artery disease (CAD) and cardiologists, surgeons and anaesthetists have shifted the emphasis onto the complex problems concerning CAD. The acquisition of skill and knowledge has minimized mortality and morbidity of patients undergoing myocardial revascularization and several authors report a low operative mortality (1-3%) (1-5).
The reported results of mitral valve replacement (MVR) are not so favourable despite longer experience in the surgical treatment of this disease (6, 7). Because of the varying socioeconomical background of the different studies, the results may have been influenced by the different aims of investigators and this could explain their variability (8-12). In a recent review (13) concerning a large series of unselected patients undergoing MVR, an operative mortality of 10,3% was reported, stressing the need for a proper evaluation of the etiological and pathological abnormalities observed in mitral valve disease.

A great amount of research (12, 14-20) has been done to detect determinants of hospital outcome and long term survival of these patients in order to set the appropriate timing for surgery and provide valid guidelines in minimizing perioperative mortality and morbidity. Deciding the appropriate time for surgery is quite well settled: the functional clinical status and valvular lesions are the determinants:

- functional class (NYHA): III - IV

- valve lesion:

  moderately severe

valve orifice	0,5 - 1 cm^2/m^2
regurgit. fraction	< 40 - 60%

severe

valve orifice < 0,5 cm^2/m^2

regurgit.fraction > 60%

The evaluation of mitral valve disease is not only determined by the type and degree of MV lesion, but also by the pathological and functional involvement of the myocardium. In rheumatic and degenerative MV lesions, advanced cardiac failure is the determinant of operative mortality (13, 21, 22).

Mitral valve lesions may develop in coronary artery disease (CAD): mitral regurgitation in CAD may occur acutely during myocardial infarction. It may become chronic due to papillary muscle rupture, chordal rupture, scarring of papillary muscle or left ventricular aneurysm; this is relatively rare and is usually seen in severe CAD with a poor ejection fraction (23, 24). The use of therapy which affects preload and afterload, with or without balloon pumping, may be helpful in stabilizing cardiovascular conditions before surgery. Surgical outcome is dependent on ventricular dysfunction and on the degree of myocardial revascularization (25). In these patients myocardial ischaemia is a determinant of myocardial failure.

Rheumatic or degenerative MV disease may be associated with CAD; the extent of CAD may affect the surgical outcome together with the severity of cardiac failure (26, 27): in these patients myocardial ischaemia exacerbates myocardial failure.

In addition, we have to consider patients who develop pulmonary artery hypertension (PAH), patients suffering from acute bacterial endocarditis and patients undergoing emergency operations.

The development of PAH frequently complicates MV disease and may significantly influence prognosis (28-33). The type of dominant MV lesion does not seem to significantly influence the preoperative pulmonary vascular resistance (PVR). Effective preoperative evaluation of PAH and of right and left ventricular function would be possible if we could extrapolate haemodynamic data in a supposedly similar condition in a normal valve.

In our experience in patients who have undergone MVR, pulmonary artery hypertension has not been a determinant of surgical outcome. Eleven patients with severe PAH ($56 < PAP < 86$ torr.; $3,5 < PVRI < 11$ U.

Wood) had a good postoperative course and 100% survival one year after surgery. Ten months after surgery all but three patients had developed an important reduction of pulmonary artery pressure (PAP) and of pulmonary vascular resistance index (PVRI).
Predictive values of postoperative PVR and PAP have not been recognized in this series of patients: right atrial pressure, wedge pressure, pulmonary artery pressure, pulmonary vascular resistance, total systemic resistance, cardiac index, intrapulmonary shunt and functional class have not given useful information. However, three patients without postoperative changes of PAP and PVRI, showed only a poor reduction of PAP and PVRI preoperatively during infusion of vasodilators (nitroglycerin, nitroprusside). Lung biopsy in these three patients showed important vascular lesions (III degree of the Heath Edwards' classification), in the remaining patients less important lesions were observed (I or II degree only, see fig. 1)

Acute infective endocarditis can be characterized by:

- extension of the infection from the valve to the mural endocardium,
- myocardial infarction (coronary embolization) not always detectable on the ECG,
- focal infective myocarditis,
- toxic and metabolic myocarditis.

Patients undergoing emergency operation have a higher mortality than those undergoing elective operations. Myocardial protection has improved survival but not in emergency cases, probably because these patients have a greater decrease of myocardial reserve and because cardioplegia can only protect and not renew myocardium. Further actuarial and pathophysiological observations which help to predict the disease course, will provide improved criteria for surgical treatment (34). The technical improvements in the surgical repair of MV suggests not to delay surgery, especially in young patients in class II. A wider surgical indication is also supported by the development of new techniques of cardiopulmonary bypass: haemodilution, no blood primes, mild hypothermia, myocardial protection and more and more advanced oxygenators. These have made cardiopulmonary bypass a relatively safe technique.

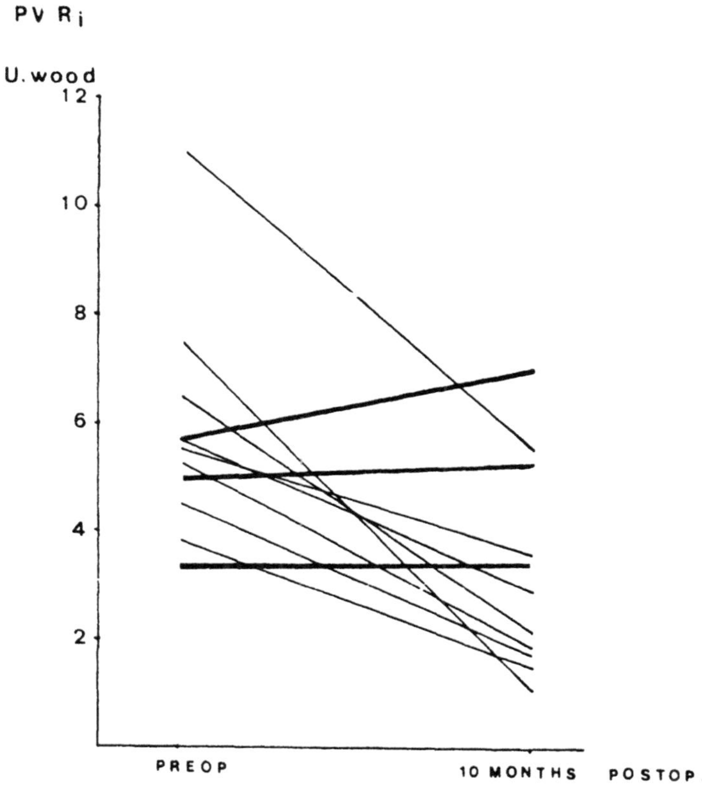

PVR_i CHANGES AFTER MVR. IN 11 PTS. WITH PAH

Mitral valve disease affects the ventricular myocardium in different ways. In mitral stenosis (MS) the right ventricle is more affected than the left ventricle. In mitral regurgitation (MR) both left and right ventricles are involved: increased thickness of the myocardial wall either alone or associated with ventricular dilatation compensates for the chronic volume and pressure overload.

At present preoperative evaluation of patients undergoing MVR is achieved by:

- assessment of the functional state of the myocardium
- assessment of "general health".

Assessment of the functional state of the myocardium

Several investigations (invasive and non-invasive) are available for this purpose.

Functional Class (NYHA) is well related to the degree of anatomical valvular abnormality (stenosis or insufficiency); class III and IV are correlated to a valve area < 2 cm^2 and to myocardial dysfunction and cardiac arrhythmias. A very important advanced functional disability (class IV) is present in patients with a severe hemodynamic deterioration (cardiac index < 2 $l/min/m^2$) and/or PAH.

ECG: reveals rhythm disturbances, ventricular hypertrophy, strain, myocardial ischaemia and previous myocardial infarction.

Chest X ray: postero anterior and lateral films show the size and the shape of the heart (cardiothoracic ratio), atria and great vessels. The degree of vascularization of the lung fields is clearly defined and confirms clinical observations. The state of pulmonary vasculature, expressed by the size of pulmonary arteries, the degree of upper lobe blood diversion and the peripheral vascularization, give good information on pulmonary hypertension and suggest further invasive and/or non-invasive investigations.

The degree of pulmonary venous congestion and pleural effusions are both indicators of poor myocardial reserve.

Echocardiography: mono- and bidimensional ECHO have considerably enhanced our diagnostic capacities in exploring MV and the quantitative assessment of heart chambers. It can explore the mitral orifice. In addition, pulsed Doppler detects turbulence and provides complementary information of mitral regurgitation on a semiquantitative basis (35). Endocarditic vegetations on the leaflets are well detected by this non-invasive approach. M and B mode ECHO provide valuable data on ventricular diameters, contractility and ejection fraction (EF). Akinesia or dyskinesia as a result of acute or chronic myocardial infarction are also easily detectable.

Radionuclide angiography provides a practical means for serial assessment of the status of left and right ventricular dimensions and function. The left ventricle's response to isometric exercise can easily be quantified by these non-invasive methods and offers the possibility of monitoring the ventricular response to afterload stress.

Cardiac catheterization. If non-invasive diagnostic means are not enough to clarify the diagnosis, a hemodynamic study may provide further information. A better understanding of the hemodynamics of MV disease and ventricular function is accomplished by quantitative angiographic techniques.

Coronary artery angiography provides good anatomical knowledge of the extent of the coronary artery disease and is mandatory for decision making and surgical approach. We believe that coronary artery angiography is advisable in all mitral valve patients older than 40 years about to undergo surgery. Recognition of coronary artery disease, even if asymptomatic, with the possibility of coronary artery bypass grafting done in association with mitral valve replacement, may improve surgical outcome of these patients.

All these invasive and non-invasive investigations have clearly improved the estimation of the functional state of the myocardium pre-and postoperatively (14, 18, 21, 36-39). However, by examining actuarial and pathophysiologic observations no single measurement alone can predict the surgical outcome. Only a careful measurement of the ratio of end-systolic stress to end-systolic volume index (40) may reflect the myocardial derangement and provide useful information about cardiac reserve.
This hemodynamic LV function evaluation is useful in patients with mitral regurgitation (MR) and should also be applied to right ventricular function. In patients with MS, who usually show normal left ventricular function, a precise right ventricular function evaluation is mandatory in predicting surgical outcome. Right ventricular function is abnormal in most patients with MV disease; this is chiefly due to inappropriate wall stress and a depressed inotropic response often leading to tricuspid regurgitation.

Assessment of "general health"

A detailed medical history and a physical examination directed towards the functional evaluation of all the subsystems are the first steps in appreciating "general health". Previous illnesses and associated illness like gastrointestinal disturbances, urinary tract infections, intermittent claudication, TIA, diabetes, hypertension, are important but not determinant of surgical outcome, rarely affecting postoperative morbidity.

Renal function should be assessed in detail in cases of inappropriately high blood urea levels associated with the clinical and cardiac condition (heart failure and high doses of diuretics); correct perioperative medical management is essential to avoid worsening of renal failure.

Severe pulmonary disease is associated with approximately twice the mortality after MV surgery; whether the concomitant pulmonary dysfunction causes increased perioperative mortality, or the pulmonary dysfunction merely is indicative of a more severe valve and/or myocardial disease, cannot be determined. Clearly patients scheduled for MVR who also have severe pulmonary dysfunction are at extremely high risk.

It is our opinion that in the preoperative assessment of the "general health" of patients undergoing MVR, two clinical conditions are the main determinants of the surgical outcome:

- preoperative liver failure (13)
- advanced malnutrition (41) i.e. cardiac cachexia.

Preoperative liver failure is not uncommon in advanced cardiac failure with prolonged systemic venous congestion and in patients who have tricuspid valve disease following right ventricular dilatation.

Liver disease is indicated by abnormal liver function tests and coagulation disorders which do not resolve when the cardiovascular status is improved; in these cases hepatic scintigraphy reveals the extent of liver damage.

Advanced malnutrition (cardiac cachexia) is a late feature of advanced cardiac failure: multiorgan failure and socioeconomical and psychological factors exacerbate this ominous clinical condition which results in a poor defence against infection and the stress of surgery. Intensive preoperative therapy and parenteral nutrition are mandatory.

We consider that a surgical approach is inadvisable in patients suffering from advanced liver disease and in patients exhibiting severe malnutrition not responding to an adequate intensive preoperative treatment.

REFERENCES

1. Cosgrove DM, Loop FD, Sheldon WC: Results of myocardial revascularization: a 12 years experience. Circulation 65 (suppl II): 37, 1982.
2. Lawrie GM, Morris GC: Survival with coronary artery bypass surgery in specific patient groups. Circulation 65 (suppl II): 43, 1982.
3. Takaro T, Hultgren HN, Lipton MJ, Detre KM and participants: VA cooperative study for coronary occlusive disease. II. Subgroup with significant left main lesions. Circulation 54 (suppl III): 107, 1976.
4. European coronary surgery study groups: Prospective randomized study of coronary artery bypass surgery in stable angina pectoris: a progress report on survival. Circulation 65 (suppl II) 67, 1982.
5. Merli M, Di Biase AM, Paleari G, Fontana F, Cattani C: L'infarto miocardico acuto peroperatorio. Atti Giornata di studio in Cardioanestesia. Bologna, 1984.
6. Lillehei CW, Gott VL, Dewall RA, Varco RL: The surgical treatment of stenotic or regurgitant lesions of the mitral and aortic valves by direct vision utilizing a pump-oxygenator. J. Thorac. Surg. 35, 154, 1958.
7. Merendino KA, Thomas GI, Jesseph JE, Herron PV, Wintersheid LC, Vetto RR: The open correction of rheumatic mitral regurgitation and/or stenosis. Ann. Surg. 150, 5, 1959.
8. Mullen JL, Buzby GP, Waldman MT, Gertner MH, Hobbs CL, Rosato EF: Prediction of operative mortality by preoperative nutritional assessment. Surg. Forum. 30, 80, 1979.
9. Leroy G, De Riberolles CH, Lecompte Y, Escande G, Marchand M, Neveux JY, Hazan E: Mortalitè perioperatoire actuelle des remplacements valvulaires. Arch. Mal. Coeur. 74, 3, 1981.
10. Jamieson WRE, Donder J, Munro AJ, Janusz MT, Burgess JJ, Miyagishima RR, Gerein AN, Allen P: Cardiac valve replacement in the elderly: a review of 320 consecutive cases. Circulation 64 (suppl II): 117, 1981.
11. Cohn LH, Koster JK Jr., Van Deventer S, Collins J Jr: The in-hospital risk of replacement of dysfunctional M and Ao Valves. Circulation (suppl I): 153, 1982.
12. Salomon NW, Stinson EB, Griepp RB: Patient related risk factors as predictors of results following isolated mitral valve replacement. Ann. Thorac. Surg. 24, 519, 1977.
13. Scott WC, Haverich A, Miller DC: Determinants of operative mortality in 1329 patients undergoing mitral valve replacement. Circulation 70 (suppl II): 238, 1984.
14. Kennedy JW, Doces JG, Stewart DK: Left ventricular function before and following surgical treatment of mitral valve disease. Am. Heart. J. 97, 592, 1979.

15. Bonchek LI: Indications for surgery of the mitral valve. Am. J. Cardiol. 46, 159, 1980.
16. Rapaport E: Natural history of aortic and mitral valve disease. Am. J. Cardiol. 35, 221, 1972.
17. Schuler G, Peterson KL, Johonson A: Tempora response of left ventricle performance to mitral valve surgery. Circulation 59, 1218, 1979.
18. Hammermeister KE, Fisher L, Kennedy JW, Samuels S, Dodge HT: Prediction of late survival in patients with mitral valve disease from clinical, hemodynamic and quantitative variables. Circulation 57, 341, 1978.
19. Ross J Jr: Left ventricular function and the timing of surgical treatment in valvular heart disease. Ann. Int. Med. 94, 498, 1981.
20. Murphy ES, Kloster FE: Late results of valve replacement surgery: I. Clinical and hemodynamic results. Mod. Concepts Cardiovasc. Dis. 48, 53, 1979.
21. Appelbaum A, Kouchoukos NT, Blackstone EH, Kirklin JW: Early risks of open heart surgery for mitral valve disease. Am. J. Cardiol. 37, 201, 1976.
22. Syracuse DC, Bowman FO Jr, Malm JR: Prosthetic valve reoperations. Factors influencing early and late survival. J. Thorac. Cardiovasc. Surg. 77, 346, 1979.
23. Gahl K, Sutton R, Pearson M, Caspari P, Lairet A, McDonald L: Mitral regurgitation in coronary heart disease. Br. Heart J. 39, 13, 1977.
24. DiSesa VJ, Cohn LH, Collings JJ Jr, Koster JK, VanDeventer S: Determinants of operative survival following combined mitral valve replacement and coronary revascularization. Ann. Thorac. Surg. 34, 482, 1982.
25. Balu V, Hershowitz S, Zaki Masud AR, Bhayana JN, Dean DC: Mitral regurgitation in coronary artery disease. Chest 81, 550, 1982.
26. Hammermeister KE, Kennedy JW: Predictors of surgical mortality in patients undergoing direct myocardial revascularization. Circulation 50 (suppl II): 112. 1974.
27. Loop FD, Berrettoni JN, Pichard A: Selection of the candidate for myocardial revascularization: a profile of high risk based on multivariate analysis. J. Thorac. Cardiovasc. Surg. 69, 40, 1975.
28. Friedman WF, Heiferman MF: Clinical problems of postoperative pulmonary vascular disease. Am. J. Cardiol. 50, 631, 1982.
29. MacKinnon J, Wade EB, Vicker CFH: Mitral stenosis with very high pulmonary vascular resistance and atypical features. Br. Heart J. 18, 449, 1956.
30. Ward C, Hancock BW: Extreme pulmonary hypertension caused by mitral valve disease. Br. Heart J. 37, 74, 1975.
31. Zener JC, Nancock EW, Shymway NE, Harrison DC: Regression of extreme pulmonary hypertension after mitral valve surgery. Am. J. Cardiol. 30, 820, 1972.
32. Cevese PG, Gallucci V, Valfre C, Giacomin A, Mazzucco A, Casarotto D: Pulmonary hypertension in mitral valve surgery. J. Cardiovasc. Surg. 21, 7, 1980.
33. Braunwald E, Braunwald NS, Ross J, Morrow AG: Effects of mitral valve replacement on the pulmonary vascular dynamics of patients with pulmonary hypertension. N. Engl. J. Med. 273, 509, 1965.
34. Peterson KL, Tajimi T: The timing of surgical intervention in chronic mitral regurgitation. In: Duran C, Angell WW, Johnson AD, Oury JH: Recent progress in mitral valve disease. Butterworth, 1984.

35. Veyrat C, Kalmanson D, Bas S, Abitbol G, Manin JP: New indices for assessing the severity of mitral regurgitation. Br. Heart J. 51, 130, 1983.
36. Urschel CW, Covell JW, Sonnenblick EH, Ross J Jr, Braunwald E: Myocardial mechanics in aortic and mitral valvular regurgitation: the concept of instantaneous impendance as a determinant of the performance of the intact heart. J. Clin. Invest. 56, 56, 1968.
37. Sagwa K: The end systolic pressure-volume relation of the ventricle: definition, modifications and clinical use. Circulation 63, 1223, 1981.
38. McGregor DC, Covell JV, Mahler F, Dilly RB, Ross J Jr: Relations between afterload, stroke volume and descending limb of Starling' curve. Am. J. Physiol. 216, 1097, 1974.
39. Schuler G, Peterson K, Hohnson A, Francis G, Dennish G, Utley J, Daily P, Ashburn W, Ross J Jr: Temporal response of left ventricular performance to mitral valve surgery. Circulation 59, 1218, 1979.
40. Carabello BA, Nolan SP, Lockhart B: Assessment of preoperative left ventricular function in patients with mitral regurgitation: Value of the end-systolic wall stress to end-systolic volume ratio. Circulation 64, 1212, 1981.
41. Pittman JG, Cohen P: The pathogenesis of cardiac cachexia. N. Engl. J. Med. 271, 403, 1964.

THE USE OF INVASIVE MONITORING TECHNQIUES IN CARDIAC SURGERY

Theodore H. Stanley, M.D.

Invasive monitoring is the product of almost 20 years of intensive technological development of devices and approaches applicable in the operating room and critical care unit. Most anesthesiologists think of pulmonary artery catheter and placement of catheters in one or more arteries as invasive monitoring. Actually invasive monitoring also includes the use of the esophageal stethoscope, urinary bladder catheter, probes placed in or near the endotracheal tube to measure inspired and end-expired gases, temperature sensitive catheters placed in the rectum, esophagus, nasal pharanyx or other orifaces, needles with pressure transducers or electrodes sensitive to changes in gas tensions, electrolytes and proteins placed in tissues, arteries or veins, electrodes placed next to or underneath the conjunctiva of the eye designed to measure PaO_2 and $PaCO_2$, and numerous other evolving methodologies aimed at recording physiologic and pharmacologic information.

Much attention has recently been paid to esophageal catheters that can monitor cardiac function. One of the most exciting of these approaches has been transesophageal two-dimensional echocardiography. This approach allows analysis of cardiac volume, contractility and motion and should prove to be an important aid in supplementing other more usually used (pulmonary and systemic arterial catheters) techniques of analyzing hemodynamics for moment-to-moment clinical cardiac assessment.

The most controversial and popular of the invasive monitoring devices ever employed has been the pulmonary artery (PA) catheter. Perhaps its popularity, availability and relative ease of use is a partial cause of the controversies that surround this instrument. It is clear that the catheter is exceedingly valuable in virtually every cardiac patient coming to operation. The reasons for this are obvious and will be discussed in greater depth. However in our cost-effecttive world, the value of routine placement of the pulmonary artery catheter in all patients and when the insertion should take place have been the focus of great attention in the last few years. This discussion will focus on some of the pros and cons of these arguments.

Of what value is a PA catheter prior to induction of anesthesia? Proponents of preinduction PA catheter placement feel that obtaining hemodynamic values prior to induction allows for optimal patient management. However most (if not all) of the information provided by a PA catheter is already available from the patient's cardiac catheterization report. This information usually includes ejection fraction, left ventricular end-diastolic pressure, cardiac output, the nature, number and degree of diseased coronary artery vessels and areas of ventricular dyskinesia. In those patients with an ejection fraction greater than 0.50 and without ventricular dysynergy, measurements of central venous pressure provide a reliable estimate of left ventricular filling pressure, eliminating the need for a PA catheter.[1] In patients with an ejection fraction less than 0.40 or ventricular dysynergy, a PA catheter provides better estimates of left ventricular filling pressure than measurement of central venous pressure, but the information must be critically evaluated.[1]

The measurement most heavily relied upon by clinicians to reflect left ventricular end-diastolic pressure (LVEDP) is the pulmonary capillary wedge pressure (PCWP). This variable also provides an estimate of left ventricular end diastolic volume.[2-5] However PCWP is not a reliable reflection of LVEDP. PCWP and LVEDP are similar in patients with normal cardiovascular dynamics but not necessarily so in patients with ischemic myocardial disease or left ventricular hypertrophy secondary to any cause.[3,4,6-8] In patients presenting for open heart surgery left ventricular compliance is frequently decreased by acute ischemia, prior myocardial infarction and hypertrophy. The noncompliant left ventricle is more dependent on atrial contraction for ventricular filling, and results in a higher LVEDP which is not reflected in the PCWP.[6-8] In these situations measurements of PCWP underestimate LVEDP. Thus a single PCWP measurement obtained prior to induction in these patients will frequently be misleading and could lead to inappropriate therapy. Furthermore, construction of Starling curves with a PCWP that underestimates LVEDP will suggest better left ventricular curves than actually exist. Whether preinduction PA catheter placement provides more information concerning a patient's cardiovascular status than cardiac catheterization data and clinical assessment (neck vein distention, gallops, rales, orthostatic hypotension, urine output) has not been explored and is therefore unknown.

Some clinicians and medical writers suggest that measurement and correction of abnormal cardiovascular variables via use of iontropic agents or vasodilators immediately prior to induction of anesthesia represents superior, modern anesthetic care. Unfortunately, supporters of this approach are unable to provide data that indicate correction of hemodynamic values prior to anesthetic induction improves outcome after open heart procedures. In a study in patients with poor left ventricular function presenting for coronary artery bypass grafting (CABG), Wynands et al.[9] showed that the mean LVEDP was 29 torr and PCWP was 22 torr.

These investigators found that in spite of no pharmacological intervention, patients were able to have anesthesia induced (using high doses of a potent narcotic) without hemodynamic alterations throughout the entire study period (the entire operation).

Proponents of preinduction PA catheterization feel that obtaining preinduction hemodynamic values allows a more rational selection of the "best anesthetic approach" for induction and maintanence of anesthesia. These proponents feel that it is worth the effort and time to obtain additional hemodynamic information (PCWP, cardiac outputs in triplicate, etc.) to help guide their anesthetic induction. However, anesthetic induction for the large majority of open heart and major vascular surgical procedures usually involves the use of one of the new synthetic narcotics (fentanyl and sufentanil). Results from many studies using these agents for induction of anesthesia have shown the process to be characteristically fast and hemodynamically uneventful. Cumulative data from eleven recently published studies (239 subjects) in patients with reasonably good left ventricular function undergoing CABG after induction with fentanyl, sufentanil or alfentanil reveal minimal or no changes in heart rate, blood pressure, cardiac output, the ECG tracing or pulmonary capillary wedge pressure.[10-20] Indeed, virtually all measured cardiovascular parameters were unchanged in all these studies.

There is less data available in patients with little or no ventricular reserve but the results are similar. Wynands and colleagues[9] studied patients with poor left ventricular function (ejection fraction less than 0.3, left ventricular end diastolic pressure greater than 20 torr and significant dyskinesia) who were given 30 ug/kg fentanyl for induction of anesthesia. They found no change in any hemodynamic variable during induction or following tracheal intubation. In another study these same investigators evaluated patients with moderate to severe left ventricular impairment (NYHA classification of III and IV).[21] In these patients they found that anesthetic induction with 50 ug/kg of fentanyl produced only a small decrease in systolic blood pressure (17%) which returned to baseline values following endotracheal intubation.

In patients undergoing mitral valve replacement, Stanley and Webster[22] found no significant changes in heart rate, stroke volume, cardiac output, peripheral vascular resistance and mean arterial and central venous pressures during and following induction of anesthesia with 11 $\pm$ 3 ug/kg of fentanyl and after endotracheal intubation. In a similar investigation Bovill et al.[23] compared fentanyl, sufentanil and alfentanil for induction of anesthesia in 60 patients with various forms of valvular heart disease. They found no changes in hemodynamics or ECG evidence of myocardial ischemia during or after the induction-intubation sequence.

Preinduction hemodynamic abnormalities can be a direct result of the insertion of a PA catheter. Placement of a PA catheter in unanesthetized patients can produce significant stimulation of the cardiovascular system.[24-25] Lunn et al.[24] evaluated PA catheter insertion in awake and anesthetized patients undergoing CABG or valve replacement operations. All patients were premedicated with 10 mg diazepam orally, 0.1 mg/kg of morphine and 0.5 mg of scopalamine intramuscularly, and all were judged adequately premedicated upon arrival to the operating room. In spite of continued verbal assurance, the use of local anesthetics and appropriate mechanical maneuvers, these authors found that systolic blood pressure and heart rate became significantly increased above baseline values in unanesthetized groups during implantation of the catheters. In contrast, patients in groups that were anesthetized did not experience changes in any cardiovascular variable. Four patients (out of forty) in the unanesthetized groups complained of angina and three had ST wave depression greater than 1 mm requiring treatment with oral nitroglycerin. DeLange and co-workers[25] studied patients about to undergo CABG or valve replacement operations who were heavily premedicated with lorazepam (0.08 mg/kg) and atropine (0.1 mg/15kg) and had a PA catheter inserted via the basilic or cephalic vein prior to induction of anesthesia. They found insertion of the PA catheter resulted in an increase in systolic arterial blood pressure in all groups and an increase in heart rate in patients about to have a CABG operation who were not receiving beta blockers. Two patients (out of 84) had angina and significant ST wave depression on the ECG.

A recent study by Slogoff and Keats[26] looked for perioperative myocardial ischemia in patients scheduled for CABG operations. The patients were given their usual beta blockers and nitrates preoperatively and were moderately or heavily premedicated. These investigators found that 18% of patients (182 out of 1023) arrived in the operating room with new ischemic ECG changes. This suggests that the anxiety and/or stress associated with transportation to the operating room and/or insertion of a venous catheter can in themselves result in serious problems. One can only wonder what the incidence of myocardial ischemia would have been if a PA catheter had been inserted prior to induction of anesthesia.

With adequate premedication and perhaps additional intravenous sedation (administered in the operating room) it is possible to insert a PA catheter without evidence of ischemia.[27-29] However the degree of central nervous system depression required can produce respiratory depression. Quintin[27] compared arterial blood gases obtained the day before CABG surgery with those sampled after PA catheter placement (prior to induction of anesthesia). They showed an increase in $PaCO_2$ from 39 torr to 45 torr and a decrease in PaO_2 from 76 torr to 69 torr. Thus the generous preoperative medication given to blunt stress responses before induction of anesthesia may pose a risk to the patient with marginal respiratory and cardiac reserve. Futhermore, sedated patients often experience hypoxemia and hypercarbia secondary to rebreathing associated with placement of drapes over their face.[30-31]

Despite lack of data, many clinicians continue to place PA catheters prior to induction of anesthesia. What motivates them to use this unnecessary and potentially dangerous crutch is unclear, since the placement of a PA catheter in unanesthetized patients needlessly provides ideal conditions for increased cardiovascular stimulation and myocardial ischemia. Evidence from many studies utilizing modern anesthetic induction agents indicates that anesthesia can be initiated rapidly and maintained uneventfully without the need of a PA catheter. Changes in hemodynamics are generally minimal, usually restricted to heart rate and blood pressure, and easily managed with usual ECG and blood pressure monitoring. Placement of a PA catheter following induction of anesthesia eliminates the risk of stress induced myocardial ischemia and allows for catheterization to proceed under more ideal and controlled conditions.

In spite of this author's fundamental belief that the PA catheter is rarely necessary for "induction of anesthesia" if a skilled anesthetist is in charge of the induction, it is fair to say that many other clincian investigators believe differently. Indeed, several reports have alluded to the benefits of pulmonary artery monitoring prior to the induction of anesthesia. In patients with left main coronary artery stenosis, Moore et al.[32] showed that preoperative PA catheter placement allowed aggressive pharmacologic interventions to optimize cardiac function, vascular tone, and volume. They suggested that this approach was at least partly responsible for a decrease in operative mortality from 20% to 3.5%. Similarly, Whittemore and co-workers[33] had no perioperative deaths in a group of 110 patients undergoing aortic aneurysm repair. They believe this notable record was partially attributed to perioperative maintenance of optimal preload and ventricular function, guided by rigorous use of the PA catheter.[33] Finally, Rao et al.[34] recently reported a significant reduction in the incidence of perioperative reinfarction in patients with ischemic heart disease undergoing non-cardiac surgery when compared to historical controls.[35] An important factor thought to contribute to this improved outcome was the aggressive use of invasive hemodynamic monitoring during the perioperative period. All patients had PA catheters placed prior to anesthetic induction. Hemodynamic abnormalities were corrected with volume replacement and rapidly acting vasoactive drugs before undergoing anesthesia. With the help of pulmonary artery monitoring, cardiovascular function was optimally maintained throughout induction and the rest of the perioperative period. Although the precise role of the PA catheter was not conclusively established, the authors speculated that it played an important role.

Other authors have attempted to show that clinical skill and experience combined with information obtained from less invasive monitors is not sufficient to diagnose and treat perioperative hemodynamic abnormalities. Waller and colleagues[36] found when experienced cardiac anesthesiologist were blinded to PA catheter measurements and their derived indices, severe abnormalities in pulmonary capillary wedge pressure (PCWP), cardiac index, and systemic vascular resistance went unnoticed 65% of the time. Thirty-four percent of these abnormalities occurred during induction. In all of these cases the anesthesiologist had to be notified of these changes so that appropriate treatment could be provided.

Authors who argue for the pre-anesthetic implantation of PA catheters state that while in ideal conditions patients should arrive in the operating room in their best possible medical condition, it often does not happen that way. Pre-operative patient history, physical examinations, and laboratory tests may not suffice to diagnose abnormalities of cardiovascular function. They maintain that astute clinicians must use the PA catheter immediately prior to anesthetic induction to detect previously unrecognized ischemia and acute abnormalities in preload and in ventricular function. Del Guercio et al.[37] described preoperative hemodynamic profiles obtained from PA and arterial cannulas in a group of 148 patients, age 65 or over, who had been declared fit for surgery by standard medical evaluation. Nearly all had some circulatory derangements and twenty-three percent had advanced deficits in cardiopulmonary function that did not respond to treatment. These abnormalities rendered them unacceptable risks for major surgery so an alternate mode of therapy was provided. Unsuspected chronic lung disease was disclosed in 12 patients who had marked elevations in their pulmonary vascular resistance (PVR). Many fell in a group that benefitted from physiologic "fine tuning" prior to anesthetic induction. Thirteen patients, who had pulmonary capillary wedge pressures greater than 15 mmHg and a low cardiac index required treatment with ionotropic agents before induction. In those patients that were hypovolemic, the PA catheter allowed close monitoring of their Frank-Starling Curve during controlled volume expansion.

In a similar study, Babu et al.[38] looked at a group of elderly patients with peripheral vascular disease. The PA catheter revealed abnormalities in preload (26.7%), and left ventricular function (40%) which were not found by conventional methods of clinical evaluation. In the group with depressed ventricular function, 13 patients required ionotropic support, ten patients needed afterload reduction, and seven patients required combinations of change in preload, ionotropic therapy, and afterload reduction. Though only general surgical patients were studied, both of these reports demonstrated that patients with atherosclerotic heart disease can benefit from PA catheter placement prior to anesthetic induction.

Some feel that cardiac catheterization data may be of limited value because it is often performed weeks to months in advance of surgery. Significant changes in cardiovascular function can occur during this interval. Furthermore, anesthetic drugs alter cardiovascular function differently in different patients. For instance, Balasaraswathi et al.[39] found that patients with elevated left ventricular end diastolic pressure respond to N_2O with decreases in cardiac output and increases in systemic vascular resistance while patients with normal left ventricular function (LVF) have no hemodynamic alterations. Similar results have been found with diazepam.[40] Etomidate, an induction agent with little or no effect on hemodynamics in patients with normal LVF, causes significant decreases of 12-19% in blood pressure and 13% in cardiac index in patients with aortic and mitral valvular heart disease.[41] Clearly, patients with poor LVF respond quite differently to anesthetics than those with normal LVF. Furthermore, placement of a PA catheter prior to induction allows immediate quantitation of LVF and detection of patients likely to be more susceptible to anesthetic-induced cardiovascular depression.

The intense sympathetic stimulation of laryngoscopy and endotracheal intubation can provoke profound hemodynamic changes, especially in patients with heart disease. Tachycardia and hypertension can promptly reduce stroke volume and create an unfavorable myocardial O_2 supply/demand ratio. Recently the potent opioids, fentanyl and sufentanil, have become popular for cardiac surgery because they produce deep levels of anesthesia without cardiovascular depression or stimulation.[17,22] However, some have questioned the reliability of these agents. Waller et al.[14] showed that fentanyl in doses ranging from 50-89 ug/kg failed to consistently block the hemodynamic reponse to laryngoscopy and intubation. In another study, 5 out of 9 patients had release of myocardial lactate during tracheal intubation reflecting myocardial ischemia after high dose (100 ug/kg) fentanyl induction.[13] Hypotension frequently occurs when supplements (diazepam, N_2O) are added to fentanyl to prevent recall.[11,22]

Proponents of a pre-induction PA catheter placement state that even with "modern induction techniques", hypertension or hypotension may result during anesthetic induction and tracheal intubation. Thus, intraarterial blood pressure monitoring has become the standard of care in patients undergoing open-heart surgery. But since blood pressure is the product of cardiac output and vascular resistance, accurate interpretation of changes in blood pressure are achieved only when these additional parameters provided by the PA catheter are available. This information confidently allows appropriate interventions to help maintain cardiovascular stability and adequate organ perfusion during induction.

Early detection of myocardial ischemia is another area where the PA catheter can be beneficial. As previously mentioned, Slogoff and Keats recently confirmed the association of perioperative myocardial ischemia with postoperative myocardial infarction.[26] Barnard et al.[42] have shown standard precordial ECG leads to be of limited use in detecting sub-endocardial ischemia. One of the earliest signs of ischemia is a decrease in left ventricular compliance.[43] Kaplan has demonstrated that abnormalities in the PCWP tracing can detect ischemia earlier than standard ECG leads II and V_5.[44] Subendocardial ischemia of papillary muscles can cause acute mitral valve regurgitation resulting in increases in PCWP and development of prominent "V" waves in the PCWP tracing. Fifteen of 18 patients who developed ischemia showed changes in the PCWP tracing while only 8 patients showed ST segment change on the ECG.

Given all of the above, what is the most rational approach? I suppose the easiest answer is to insert the PA catheter before anesthesia if it will provide information that will significantly alter preanesthetic management and anesthetic induction, If it won't alter management then it should not be inserted until after induction of anesthesia.

REFERENCES

1. Mangano DT: Monitoring pulmonary arterial pressure in coronary artery disease. Anesthesiology 53:364-370, 1980

2. Kaltman AJ, Herbert WH, Conroy RJ, Kossman CE: The gradient across the pulmonary vascular bed during diastole. Circulation 34:377-384, 1966

3. Falicov RE, Resnekov L: Relationship of the pulmonary artery end-diastolic pressure to the left ventricular end-diastolic pressure in patients with and without left ventricular dysfunction. Circulation 42:65-73, 1970

4. Bouchard RJ, Gault JH, Ross J JR: Evaluation of pulmonary arterial end-diastolic pressure as an estimate of left ventricular end-diastolic pressure in patients with normal and abnormal left ventricular performance. Circulation 44:1072-1079, 1971

5. Jenkins BS, Brandley RD, Branthwaite MA: Evaluation of pulmonary arterial end-diastolic pressure as an indirect estimate of left atrial mean pressure. Circulation 42:75-83, 1970

6. Rahimtoola SH, Loeb HS, Ehsani A, Sinno MZ, Chuquimia R, Lai R, Rosen KM, Gunnar RM: Relationship of pulmonary artery to left ventricular diastolic pressures in acute myocardial infarction. Circulation 46:283-290, 1972

7. Rahimtoola SH: Left ventricular end-diastolic and filling pressures in assessment of ventricular function. Chest 63:858-860, 1973

8. Rahimtoola SH, Ehsani A, Sinno MZ, Loeb HS, Rosen KM, Gunnar RM: Left atrial transport function in myocardial infarction. Importance of its booster pump function. Am J Med 59:686-693, 1975

9. Wynands JE, Wong P, Whalley DG, Sprigge JS, Townsend GE, Patel YC: Oxygen-fentanyl anesthesia in patients with poor left ventricular function: hemodynamics and plasma fentanyl concentrations. Anesth Analg 62:476-482, 1983

10. Stanley TH, Philbin DM, Coggins CH: Fentanyl-oxygen anaesthesia for coronary artery surgery: cardiovascular and antidiuretic hormone responses. Canad Anaesth Soc J 26(3):168-172, 1979

11. Lunn JK, Stanley TH, Eisele J, Webster L, Woodward A: High dose fentanyl anesthesia for coronary artery surgery: plasma fentanyl concentrations and influence of nitrous oxide on cardiovascular responses. Anesth Analg 58:390-395, 1979

12. De Lange S, Stanley TH, Boscoe MJ: Alfentanil-oxygen anaesthesia for coronary artery surgery. Br J Anaesth 53:1291-1296, 1981

13. Sonntag H, Larsen R, Kilfiker O, Kettler D, Brockschnieder B: Myocardial blood flow and oxygen consumption during high-dose fentanyl anesthesia in patients with coronary artery disease. Anesthesiology 56:417-422, 1982

14. Waller JL, Hug CC, Nagle DM, Craver JM: Hemodynamic changes during fentanyl-oxygen anesthesia for aortocoronary bypass operation. Anesthesiology 55:212-217, 1981

15. Sprigge JS, Wynands JE, Whalley DG, Bevan DR, Townsend GE, Nathan H, Patel YC, Srikant CB: Fentanyl infusion anesthesia for aorotocoronary bypass surgery: plasma levels and hemodynamic response. Anesth Analg 61:972-978, 1982

16. de Lange S, Boscoe MJ, Stanley TH, Pace N: Comparison of sufentanil-O_2 and fentanyl-O_2 for coronary artery surgery. Anesthesiology 56:112-118, 1982

17. Sebel PS, Bovil JG: Cardiovascular effects of sufentanil anesthesia. Anesth Analg 61:115-119, 1982

18. de Lange S, Boscoe MJ, Stanley TH, de Bruijin N, Philbin DM, Coggins CH: Antidiuretic and growth hormone responses during coronary artery surgery with sufentanil-oxygen and alfentanil-oxygen anesthesia in man. Anesth Analg 61:434-438, 1982

19. Zurick AM, Urzua J, Yared JP, Estafanous FG: Comparison of hemodynamic and hormonal effects of large single-dose fentanyl anesthesia and halothane/nitrous oxide anesthesia for coronary artery surgery. Anesth Analg 61:521-526, 1982

20. Hicks HC, Mowbray AG, Yhap EO: Cardiovascular effects of and catecholamine responses to high dose fentanyl-O_2 for induction of anesthesia in patients with ischemic coronary artery disease. Anesth Analg 60:563-568, 1981

21. Quintin L, Whalley DG, Wynands JE, Morin JE, Burke J: High dose fentanyl anaesthesia with oxygen for aorto-coronary bypass surgery. Canad Anaesth Soc J 28:314-320, 1981

22. Stanley TH, Webster LR: Anesthetic requirements and cardiovascular effects of fentanyl-oxygen and fentanyl-diazepam-oxygen anesthesia in man. Anesth Analg 57:411-416, 1978

23. Bovill JG, Warren PJ, Schuller JL, van Wezel HB, Hoeneveld MH: Comparison of fentanyl, sufentanil, and alfentanil anesthesia in patients undergoing valvular heart surgery. Anesth Analg 73:1081-1086 ,1984

24. Lunn JK, Stanley TH, Webster LR, Bidwai AV: Arterial blood-pressure and pulse-rate responses to pulmonary and radial arterial catheterization prior to cardiac and major vascular operations. Anesthesiology 51:256-269, 1979

25. De Lange SS, Boscoe MJ, Stanley TH: Percutaneous pulmonary artery catheterization via the arm before anaesthesia: success rate, frequency of complications and arterial pressure and heart rate responses. Br J Anaesth 53:1167-1171, 1981

26. Slogoff S, Keats AS: Does perioperative myocardial ischemia lead to postoperative myocardial infarction? Anesthesiology 62(2):107-114, 1985

27. Quintin L, Whalley DG, Wynands JE, Morin JE: The effects of vascular catheterizations upon heart rate and blood pressure before aortocoronary bypass surgery. Canad Anaesth Soc J 28(3):244-247, 1981

28 Waller JL, Zaidan JR, Kaplan JA, Bauman DI: Hemodynamic responses to preoperative vascular cannulation in patients with coronary artery disease. Anesthesiology 56:219-221, 1982

29. Waller JL, Zaidan JR, Kaplan JA, Bauman DI: Hemodynamic effects of vascular cannulation by residents. Anesthesiology 53(2):S114, 1980

30. Weisman H, Christensen RE, Dillon JB: An air-conditioned, adjustable table frame for eye surgery. Arch Ophthal 83:448-449, 1970

31. Ramanathan S, Capan L, Chalon J, Rand PB, Klein GS, Turndorf H: Mini-environmental control under the drapes during operations on the eyes of conscious patients. Anesthesiology 48(4):286-288, 1974

32. Moore CH, Combardo TR, Allums JA, Gordon FT: Left main coronary artery stenosis: hemodynamic monitoring to reduce mortality. Ann Thorac Surg 26:445-449, 1978

33. Whittemore AD, Clowes AW, Hectman HB, Mannick JA: Aortic aneurysm repair-reduced operative mortality associated with the maintenance of optimal cardiac performance. Ann Surg 192:414-421, 1980

34. Rao TLK, Jacobs KH, El-etr AA: Reinfarction following anesthesia in patients with myocardial infarction. Anesthesiology 59:499-505, 1983

35. Stern PA, Tinker JH, Tarhan S: Myocardial reinfarction after anesthesia and surgery. JAMA 239:2566-2570, 1978

36. Waller JL, Johnson SP, Kaplan JA: Usefulness of pulmonary artery catheters during aortocoronary bypass surgery. Anesth Analg 61: 221-222, 1982

37. Louis RM, Del Guercio LRM, Cohn JP: Monitoring operative risk in the elderly. JAMA 243:1350-1355, 1980

38. Babu SC, Sharma PVP, Raciti A, Mayr CH, Elrabie NA, Clauss RH, Stahl WM, Del Guercio LRM: Monitor guided responses, operability with safety is increased in patients with peripheral vascular disease. Arch Surg 115:1384-1386, 1980

39. Balasaraswathi K, Kumar P, Rao TKL, El-etr AA: Left ventricular end-diastolic pressure as an index for nitrous oxide use during coronary artery surgery. Anesthesiology 55:708-709, 1981

40. Dauchot PJ, Staub F, Berzina L, Van Heeckeren D, MacKay W, Sirvaitis R: Hemodynamic response to diazepam: dependence on prior left ventricular end diastolic pressure. Anesthesiology 60:499-503, 1984

41. Colvin MP, Savage JM, Newland PE: Cardiorespiratory changes following induction of anaesthesia with etomidate in patients with cardiac disease. Br J Anaesth 51:551-556, 1979

42. Barnard RJ, Buckberg GD, Duncan HW: Limitations of the standard transthoracic ECG in detecting subendocardiac ischemia. Am Heart J 99:476-82, 1980

43. Rao TLK: Cardiac monitoring for the noncardiac surgical patient. Seminars in Anesthesia 2:241-250, 1983

44. Kaplan JA, Wells PH: Early diagnosis of myocardial ischemia using the PA catheter. Anesth Analg 60:789-93, 1981

INOTROPIC AGENTS / VASOACTIVE AGENTS

Hempelmann G., Seidelmayer E.

A basic knowledge in cardiovascular physiology and pharmacology is a "must" in modern anesthesiology. Flow rate, pressure and resistance are linked to each other by the law of Ohm (equation 1). Resistance is related to viscosity, radius and length (equation 2). The well known HAGEN-POISEUILLE equation (3) is indicating that the perfusion of an organ or tissue area is depending on several factors:

1. It is directly proportional to the effective pressure, which is the difference between arterial and venous pressure.
2. It is directly proportional to the radius of the vascular bed; minimal changes of the radius cause tremendous influence on flow rates.
3. It is inversely proportional to the viscosity of the blood.
4. It is inversely proportional to the length of the capillary bed - a given anatomical fact.

$$R = \frac{8 \eta l}{\pi r^4}$$

$$Q = \frac{P}{R}$$

$$Q = \frac{(P_1 - P_2) \pi r^4}{8 \eta l}$$

FIGURE 1: Basic equations

Although we know that the HAGEN-POISEUILLE equation is not strictly applicable to the circulatory system because of limitations such as long tubes, rigid walls and restrictions to laminar flow and Newtonian liquids, it gives us a fundamental approximation for therapeutic rationalisation:

1. Positive inotropic drugs increase myocardial contractility, thus increasing pressure difference and consequently flow rates.
2. Vasodilating drugs enlarge vascular radius, by which total peripheral resistance is decreased; this induces a decrease in cardiac work on one hand and improves tissue perfusion on the other hand.
3. A decrease in viscosity can improve flow rates. One has to keep in mind, however, that the systemic transport of oxygen is maximal in the hematocrit range between 35 and 45 %, when inducing hemodilution. Furthermore it is of interest, that plasma viscosity is a function of plasma protein concentration and composition. Fibrinogen can decrease flow rates more than albumin solutions, and inversely viscosity

can be reduced and microcirculation improved by means of defibrination.

In the following I would like to discuss some drugs of clinical relevance, being able to improve myocardial function either by improving inotropic state, cardiac output or blood pressure - in any event myocardial oxygen demand is increased. Furthermore, I shall mention vasodilating drugs, being of interest during an intraoperative period, when a decrease in preload, afterload, cardiac work and/or myocardial oxygen demand and an improvement in microcirculation is necessary. In most clinical situations a combination of one of the drugs of each of the two groups probably will be the most effective way of treatment.

INOTROPIC AGENTS

Positive inotropic agents are drugs, which increase myocardial contractility at a given preload and afterload. They act by increasing activator calcium ion availability. Following groups are of interest:

1. Cardiac glycosides
2. Glucagon
3. Phosphodiesterase inhibitors such as aminophylline
4. Catecholamines and their derivatives
5. New drugs: amrinone, prenalterol, ARL and others.

Cardiac glycosides

Cardiac glycosides were the first widely used positive inotropic agents. Nevertheless their exact mechanism of action still is not clear. There have been some controversial results with respect to their effects in normal and failing hearts. Today, however, it is generally accepted, that cardiac glycosides increase contractility in normal as well as in failing hearts. The following mechanisms of action are discussed:

1. Inhibition of the Na^+- K^+ - pump
2. Augmentation of the calcium-pump
3. Unknown effects on the heart
4. In addition to their cardiac effects glycosides constrict isolated arterial and venous segments.

EFFECTS OF CARDIAC GLYCOSIDES

<u>non-failing heart</u>:

- CO - (↓)
- $M\dot{V}O_2$ ↑
- TSR ↑

<u>failing heart</u>:

- CO ↑
- $M\dot{V}O_2$ (↓)
- TSR (↓)

FIGURE 2: Effects of cardiac glycosides

In the non failing heart the net hemodynamic and metabolic effects are characterized by an unchanged or slightly decreased cardiac output, an increased myocardial oxygen consumption and peripheral vasoconstriction. In cardiac failure, the increase in output by digitalis glycosides is leading to reflex withdrawal of enhanced sympathetic tone; this mechanism overrides the small vasoconstrictory effect. Therefore the net hemodynamic and metabolic effects of glycosides in cardiac failure are characterized by an increase in cardiac output, a decrease in heart rate, left ventricular filling pressure, myocardial oxygen consumption and peripheral resistance. Although the cardiovascular effects of cardiac glycosides are of advantage, their importance in the intraoperative period has decreased because of a delay in onset of action, side effects and a rather long half-life. They might be indicated, when catecholamines and vasodilating agents alone are not effective enough.

Glucagon

Although the polypeptide glucagon has been discovered already in 1923, positive inotropic effects are first described in 1960 by FARAH and TUTTLE. The exact mechanism of action is not known; like the catecholamines it causes an increase in the myocardial concentration of cyclic AMP by a stimulation of adenyl cyclase. It is interesting to realize, that there is a specific glucagon receptor.

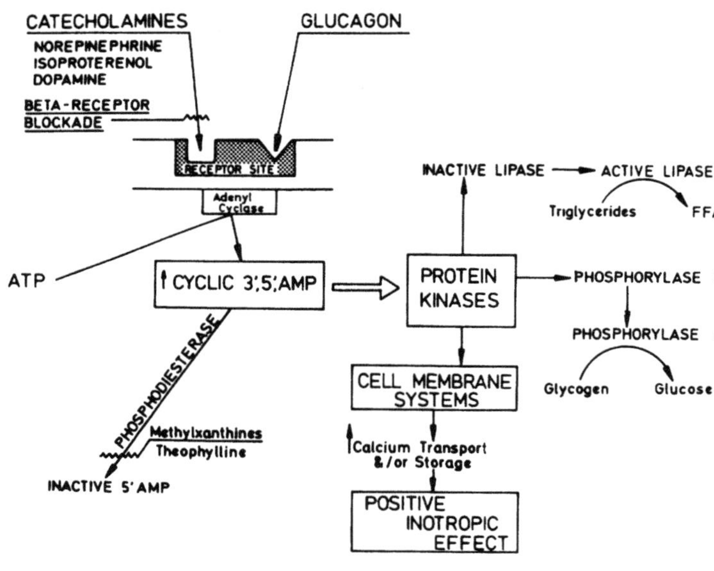

FIGURE 3: Possible mechanism of action of catecholamines and glucagon (1).

From the clinical point of view experiences with glucagon have been disappointing. In patients suffering from chronic heart failure there was almost no effect. In acute heart failure its action is limited. A bolus injection of glucagon can increase systolic and diastolic blood pressure as well as heart rate; stroke volume and cardiac output may rise, too, immediately after injection, whereas a continuous infusion of 0,06 $mg \times kg^{-1} \times h^{-1}$ has not been able to stabilize cardiovascular parameters at the initially elevated level in our patients. Only seldom there is a need for this inotropic agent - maybe at the end of extracorporeal circulation, when a patient cannot be weaned off the pump inspite of prolonged reperfusion time and administration of catecholamines, vasodilators, glucose, insulin, and optimal volume therapy, especially, when a beta-receptor-blockade might be the underlying cause for myocardial insufficiency.

Phosphodiesterase Inhibitors

Another in cardiac failure rarely used inotropic agent is aminophylline. It is mainly used in the treatment of bronchospasm and asthma. In patients suffering from these diseases it may contribute to cardiac stimulation.
Three modes of action are being discussed:

1. Inhibition of phosphodiesterase, which leads to an increase in cyclic AMP in cardiac muscle, stimulating myocardial contractility.
2. Aminophylline stimulates catecholamine release from the adrenal medulla and extra-adrenal chromaffine tissue.
3. Aminophylline has a direct effect on cell membranes, causing an increased calcium entry, which enhances contractility.

Furthermore, aminophylline dilates arteries and veins, which might cause an initial hypotension, when given intravenously. Its positive inotropic effect is rather small and of short duration; the net increase in cardiac output is primarily due to a decrease in afterload. Its positive chronotropic effect limits the indication as a cardiac stimulant.

Catecholamines and their derivatives

Undoubtedly the catecholamines and their derivatives represent the most important group of inotropic agents. Their mechanism of action is mediated by an increase in cellular cyclic AMP via adrenergic receptors and an activation of adenylcyclase activity. Cyclic AMP stimulates protein kinases and enhances calcium influx.
The most often used substances in this group are the naturally occuring epinephrine, norepinephrine and dopamine and their synthetic derivatives orciprenaline and dobutamine.Recently there have been developed further derivatives of direct and indirect sympathomimetics, for example amrinone and prenalterol, which perhaps will open new possibilities in treating cardiac failure.

	CARDIAC	VASCULAR	
Sympathomimetic agent	β_1	α	β_2
Orciprenaline(Alupent)	+++	0	+++
Epinephrine (Suprarenin)	+++	+ → ++	++ → +
Dobutamine (Dobutrex)	+++	+	+
Dopamine* (Dopamine)	++	+ → ++	+
Norepinephrine (Arterenol)	+	+++	-

FIGURE 4: Important catecholamines

But the largest clinical experience exists with the above mentioned long known and used substances, and this paper will refer only to them. The following tables show the main actions of these substances in a concise overview:

HEMODYNAMICS OF ORCIPRENALINE

- stimulation of $\underline{\beta_1}$ and $\underline{\beta_2}$ receptors
- inotropic and chronotropic effect
- CO ↑, HR ↑, (→ CO ↓), $\dot{V}_{cor}$ ↑, $M\dot{V}O_2$ ↑
- preload ↓, afterload ↓,
- if p_{diast} ↓ → $\dot{V}_{cor}$ ↓
- maldistribution of CO, ventricular ectopic beats

FIGURE 5: Hemodynamics of orciprenaline

Orciprenaline

The primary indication for orciprenaline is given by its positive chronotropic effect. In bradycardia nowadays, however, sequential pacing is preferred quite often in open cardiac surgery and also in long term treatment of severe bradycardia.

Epinephrine

Epinephrine is the drug of choice in resuscitation. In long-term inotropic therapy a decrease in renal blood flow and an increase in heart rate has limited its indication. In our hands it is still the drug of choice immediately after extracorporeal circulation because of its superb increase in contractility; this is of increasing importance since more and more patients coming for coronary bypass surgery are on calcium antagonist therapy. In higher dosages, however, a vasodilator is added for reduction of pre- and afterload to improve cardiac economy and tissue perfusion.

HEMODYNAMICS OF EPINEPHRINE

- stimulation of $\underline{\beta_1}$, $\underline{\beta_2}$ and $\underline{\alpha}$ receptors
- CO ↑, HR ↑, $\dot{V}_{cor}$ ↑, $M\dot{V}O_2$ ↑
- in larg doses → TSR ↑, arrhythmia (→ addition of vasodilator)

FIGURE 6: Hemodynamics of epinephrine

Dobutamine

A major advantage of dobutamine is its positive inotropic effect without influencing heart rate and afterload too much. In many instances it has replaced epinephrine and dopamine, the latter one especially in the postoperative period, when renal function is not compromised. For intra-operative management we still prefer epinephrine, because dobutamine is not increasing contractility and cardiac output in the same way.

HEMODYNAMICS OF DOBUTAMINE

- stimulation of $\underline{\beta_1}$, $\underline{\beta_2}$ and α receptors
- CO $\uparrow$, HR ($\uparrow$), $\dot{V}_{cor}$ $\uparrow$, $M\dot{V}O_2$ $\uparrow$
- p_{syst} $\uparrow$, p_{diast} ~, TSR ~; TPR ($\downarrow$)
- maldistribution of CO $\longrightarrow$ skeletal muscle

FIGURE 7: Hemodynamics of dobutamine

Dopamine

Dopamine certainly is a very valuable drug in the treatment of cardiovascular insufficiency. In contrast to the other catecholamines it increases renal blood flow, glomerular filtration and natriuresis. In cardiac patients with borderline renal function we administer dopamine intravenously in a dose of 200 µg|min during the intraoperative period. If a larger increase in inotropy is necessary, we add epinephrine, sometimes in combination with a vasodilator. Except of this we generally are not combining several catecholamines, because the mechanism of receptor activation may be disguised by this; one catecholamine and one vasodilator should be able to cope with most of the intraoperative destabilized hemodynamic situations. At a given filling pressure, dobutamine seems to have an advantage compared to dopamine.

HEMODYNAMICS OF DOPAMINE

- stimulation of β_1, β_2, α and dopamine receptors; dose dependent $\longrightarrow$ α receptor
- low dosage $\longrightarrow$ $V_{ren} \uparrow$, TSR $\downarrow$, CO $\uparrow$, HR $\uparrow$
- high dosage $\longrightarrow$ dominating α-stimulation, p $\uparrow$, $M\dot{V}O_2 \uparrow$
- $\longrightarrow$ ectopic beats, tachycardia

FIGURE 8: Hemodynamics of dopamine

Norepinephrine

Although norepinephrine is stimulating also β_1-receptors, its main effect relates to α-receptors, increasing total systemic resistance. At low dosage an increase in heart rate, cardiac output, blood pressure and contractility may be of advantage. Medium and higher dosages of course induce detrimental effects because of severe vasoconstriction and compromised microcirculation, reflex bradycardia and an eventual decrease in cardiac output. From the clinical point of view there might be an indication in situations with low perfusion pressure due to excessive peripheral vasodilation like in septic patients or after severe anaphylactoid reactions. It might be the only possibility to achieve a sufficient diastolic perfusion pressure. Also in patients being on the intraaortic balloon pump or during extracorporeal circulation with a too low perfusion pressure (after all other modulating mechanisms have been checked upon) there could be an indication for norepinephrine or, even more for a pure vasoconstrictor.

Calcium

A short review of some positive inotropic agents has to include calcium, although it seems to become unpopular. But an acute intraoperative decrease in blood pressure, for example after protamine application, stills seems to be an indication for a calcium bolus injection to achieve a rapid stabilisation, which, although short termed, may bridge the time until a catecholamine perfusor is started, if necessary.

HEMODYNAMICS OF NOREPINEPHRINE

- stimulation of β_1 and $\underline{\alpha}$ receptors
- CO (↑↓), HR (↓), $M\dot{V}O_2$ ↑, TSR ↑
- indications ⟶ septic shock, anaphylactoid shock, IABP

FIGURE 9: Hemodynamics of norepinephrine

The catecholamines and their derivatives share, in different degree and dose related some adverse effects: Tachycardia, increased heart work and oxygen demand are dangerous for patients with coronary heart disease. The incidence of dysrhythmias and ectopias is increased. The constriction of the small vessels raises afterload and thus heart work, decreases tissue perfusion and thus compromises organ function.
These side effects sometimes limit their usefulness and give reason to the need for substances, which are able to lower and economize heart work and improve tissue perfusion.

VASODILATORS

Vasodilating drugs are able to fullfill these therapeutic wishes. Many drugs are able to induce peripheral vasodilation by different means; sodiumnitroprusside and nitroglycerin are the two drugs, which are superior in meeting the demands of the intra- and postoperative period. Their effects are pronounced, of rapid onset and short duration and thus well controllable. The further comments will be limited to these two substances.
Both vasodilators have an effect at the arterial and venous side. Sodium nitroprusside, however, is decreasing arterial pressure much more than nitroglycerin. If a reduction in arterial impedance, afterload and blood pressure is essential, we prefer sodium nitroprusside. A preload reduction without compromising arterial pressure too much can be accomplished by nitroglycerin.

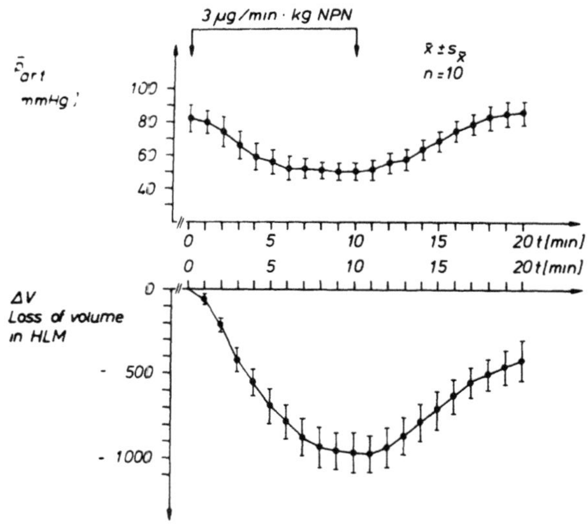

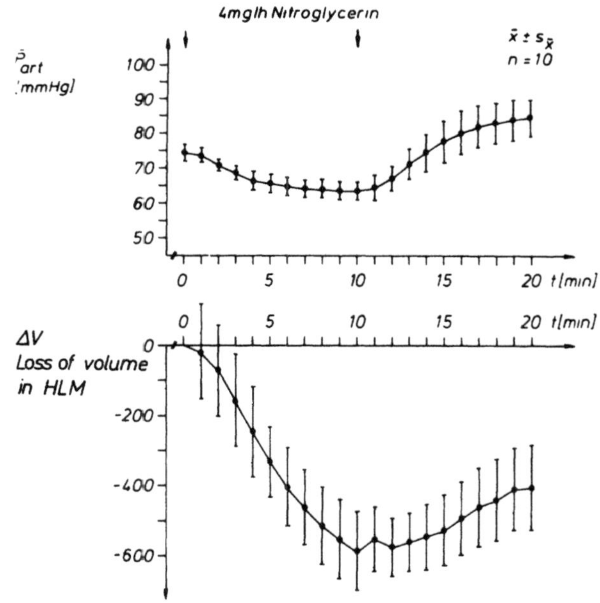

FIGURE 10 and 11: Vasodilatory effects of sodium nitroprusside (fig. 10) and nitroglycerin (fig 11) during extracorporeal circulation (from Piepenbrock S. and G. Hempelmann in (8)

The separate effects of both substances can be demonstrated during extracorporeal circulation.

Nitroglycerin is lowering arterial perfusion pressure in a moderate way, whereas venous capacitance vessels are dilated far more, as one can see from the decrease of volume in the oxygenator.
Sodium nitroprusside is decreasing arterial pressure during extracorporeal circulation more effectively, at the venous side the dilating effect is rather significant as well.

In any patient hemodynamic reactions to a vasodilator depend on the preexisting cardiovascular state. This can be illustrated by a diagram of COHN and FRANCIOSA: Small segments of preload curves (left ventricular filling pressure) are superimposed on outflow resistance curves (impedance), both being plotted against cardiac output.

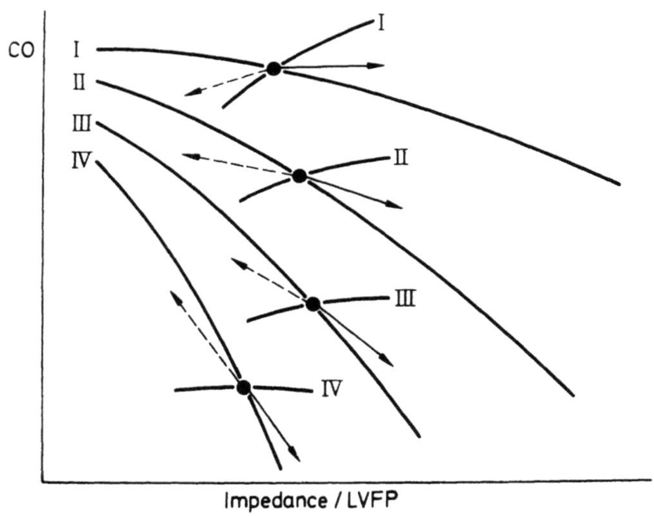

FIGURE 12: Function curves of the heart (recited from (8))

Curves I and II are normal and slightly impaired cardiac function curves. In a normal heart a preload reduction is causing a more pronounced effect than a reduction in impedance; the hemodynamic net effect is characterized by a decrease in cardiac output (dotted line). Preload and impedance curves III and IV characterize severe myocardial disease, these hearts are operating on a rather flat function curve and a markedly depressed impedance curve. In situations like this impedance reduction predominates preload effects- the hemodynamic net effect is a rise in cardiac output.

The intraoperative management of cardiovascular insufficiency can be achieved with inotropic and/or vasoactive agents. Before the application of these drugs is indicated oxygenation, ventilation, oxygen transport capacity, metabolism, blood viscosity and imbalances in electrolyte and acid-base status should be checked upon. If a normalisation of these parameters is not effective enough or possible the indication for one of the former mentioned drugs is given. The application has to be based on cardiovascular principles with respect to the present myocardial and vascular situation.

REFERENCES

1. Antonaccio MJ: Cardiovascular Pharmacology, New York, Raven Press, 1977
2. Braunwald E: Heart disease. A textbook of cardiovascular medicine, Saunders Comp. Philadelphia, London
3. Delius W, Gerlach E, Grobecker H, Kübler W: Catecholamines and the Heart, Springer,Berlin,Heidelberg, New York, 1981
4. Hurst JW et al.: The Heart, MacGraw Hill,
5. Kaplan JA: Cardiac Anesthesia, Volume 1. Clinical cardiology monographs, Grune & Stratton, New York, San Francisco, London, 1979
6. Kaplan JA: Cardiac Anesthesia, Volume 2. Cardiovascular Pharmacology, Grune & Stratton, New York, San Francisco, London, 1983
7. Prys-Roberts C: The Circulation in Anesthesia. Applied Physiology and Pharmacology, Blackwell
8. Roskamm H, Schmutziger M: Coronary Heart Surgery. Springer, Berlin, Heidelberg, New York, 1979
9. Smith LDR, Oldershaw PJ: Inotropic and Vasopressor Agents. Br.J. Anesth. 56, 767, 1984.

TECHNQIUES OF ANESTHETIC ADMINISTRATION: ARE THEY MORE IMPORTANT THAN CHOICE OF ANESTHETIC AGENT?

Theodore H. Stanley, M.D.

Modern anesthetic agents such as highly potent opioids, benzodiazepine compounds and some of the new nonbarbiturate, ultra short-acting sedative/ hypnotics have minimal effects on cardiovascular dynamics and often only modest effects on the respiratory system. As a result, traditional methods of assessing and maintaining anesthetic depth are less reliable and more difficult to master. In addition, the use of other agents including anesthetic supplements, muscle relaxants, and compounds employed by nonanesthetic personnel such as surgeons and internists may have a marked effect on respiratory and cardiac function when used concurrently with modern intravenous anesthetics. These changes focus on anesthetic technique and make technique more critical than it has ever been in the past. This discussion will focus on the subtle manouvers which are often necessary to insure that modern anesthetics are used correctly. It will identify dangerous traps such as using large bolus doses of easily applied compounds (opioids) with or without muscle relaxants which can produce virtually instantaneous anesthesia but at serious physiological and pharmacological cost. The discussion will address "clinical traps" that often occur with modern anesthetic agents and how to avoid them. The paper will use patients with cardiovascular disease, particularly coronary artery (CAD) and valvular heart disease (VHD) as illustrative examples because these patients depend on modern anesthetic agents and "ideal" techniques more than any other group. Nonetheless the principles are applicable to many if not all other patients.

Induction of Anesthesia

Perhaps the single greatest advantage of the modern high dose opioid techniques now frequently employed for patients with cardiac disease undergoing cardiac or non-cardiac operations is the ability of these agents to rapidly induce profound analgesia and anesthesia without significantly affecting cardiovascular dynamics. This is of particular importance during anesthetic induction. With large "anesthetic" doses of fentanyl and sufentanil, significant hypotension and severe bradycardia are rare. Nonetheless, some clinicians have difficulties recognizing when patients are unconscious. Occasionally patients who appear to be unconscious have vigorous eyelid reflexes which are confusing to the anesthetist inexperienced with opioids. This is quite different from inhalation anesthetics, which clearly depress all reflexes and make the end point of anesthetic induction much easier to determine.

Morphine

In order to minimize the risk of hypotension during induction of anesthesia, morphine often is administered slowly over a minimum of 10-15 min. This is accomplished most easily with the use of a 0.1% solution of morphine in either dextrose (5%) or dextrose-saline at a rate of 5-10 mg/min, with the patient breathing 100% oxygen or oxygen plus N_2O until a satisfactory level of anesthesia occurs.[1-7] The incidence of hypotension during induction also may be minimized by concurrent administration of a rapid infusion of intravenous fluids[4,7] by placing the patient in a sight Trendelenberg position[4,7] and/or by pretreatment with histamine (H_1 and H_2) receptor blockers.[8]

Induction of anesthesia usually requires 1-3 mg/kg of morphine,[1-6] depending on the patient's clinical condition, but may require larger amounts, especially in patients with reasonable cardiac reserve.[9] Since significant respiratory depression will occur before loss of consciousness in most patients, ventilatory assistance and then controlled ventilation usually is required. Often sedative/hyponotic compounds are added before or during administration of morphine to reduce opioid dosage and insure amnesia.[2,9] Once unconsciousness has been acheived, a muscle relaxant is given, the trachea is intubated, and ventilation continued with either oxygen, an air-oxygen mixture, or nitrous oxide in oxygen,[1,3] Careful observation of the patient's response to laryngoscopy and intubation can provide useful information as to the adequacy of anesthesia. Increases in blood pressure and heart rate, muscle or eyelid movement, and furrowing of the forehead all suggest an inadequate depth of anesthesia and are indications for additional morphine and/or intravenous or inhalation anesthetic supplementation before surgery commences.[7,10] Likewise, reactions to surgical stimuli usually can be treated by similar therapies or, if the patient is considered to be adequately anesthetized, with an intravenous (nitroglycerin or sodium nitroprusside) or inhalation (low concentrations of enflurane or isoflurane) vasodilator.[11]

Similar infusion techniques have been used by many clinicians and investigators to obtain anesthesia with fentanyl.[12-20] Induction of anesthesia via slow infusion of fentanyl, in contrast to infusion of morphine, usually is begun after a small dose of nondepolarizing muscle relaxant (pancuronium, 1-1.5 mg, *d*-tubocuraine, 3-4.5 mg, or metocurine, 1.0-3.5 mg) to minimize or prevent muscle rigidity. Infusion rates of fentanyl generally have ranged from 200-400 ug/min,[12,18,20,21] but the rationale for and techniques of preoperative patient preparation, premedication, anesthetic supplementation during induction and maintenance periods, determination of unconsciousness (anesthesia), muscle relaxants and doses used for endotracheal intubation, and the remainder of the operation and total doses of fentanyl have varied enormously.[7,12,13,17,19-27] Many of these differences may be attributed to the question (debate) whether fentanyl should be considered an anesthetic.[24-27] Similar questions were raised more than a decade ago, when high does of morphine were popular.[2] Unfortunately, these questions are, as yet, incompletely answered, and it is likely that the debate and enormous variety of methods of using fentanyl for complete anesthesia or as an analgesic supplement will continue.

Some clinicians feel it is quicker, easier, and more rational to infuse a single large, precalculated bolus dose of fentanyl (50-100 ug/kg), usually with a large bolus dose of pancuronium (0.1- 0.12 mg/kg, to minimize fentanyl-induced bradycardia) for both induction and maintenance of anesthesia.[28-37] Following this, ventilation is controlled, the trachea intubated and, within moments, the patient is ready for surgical preparation. Variations on the "bolus" technique are as numerous as the slower "infusion" approach of using fentanyl, undoubtedly for the same reasons. Bolus approaches seem less rational because they do not allow titration to effect and thus determination of each patient's individual anesthetic needs and can be associated with hemodynamic instability. Furthermore, they demand (or rather often employ) the large bolus dose of a non-depolarizing muscle relaxant which can result in unfavorable hemodyanmic changes by itself.

Sufentanil is a new fentanyl-like opioid which has recently been made available. It is probably 7-12 times as potent as fentanyl and has a terminal elimination half-life ($T_{1/2}B$) which is shorter (149 min) compared with the values reported for fentanyl which vary between 219 min and 495 min.[38-40] This difference should result in a shorter duration of action for sufentanil, particulary where high doses or repeated doses are being used. However, studies comparing anesthetic doses of sufentanil with comparable doses of fentanyl in patients undergoing coronary artery surgery have not demonstrated any clinically significant differences in recovery from anesthesia or time to extubation.[41,42]

Because very large doses of sufentanil produce minimal hemodynamic change in dogs,[43] sufentanil has been suggested as an alternative opioid anesthetic to fentanyl.[43,41] Some studies now have been carried out evaluating this agent as a complete anesthetic.[41] Sufentanil 15 ug/kg, with air/O_2 as an anesthetic for cardiac surgery, produced no significant changes in cardiovascular dynamics.[44] There was also a lesser incidence of hypertension related to sternotomy (10% of patients required vasodilator therapy) using sufentanil 15 ug/kg than fentanyl 70 ug/kg (50% requried vasodilators). In a study comparing fentanyl (mean total dose 122 ug/kg), with sufentanil (mean total dose 12.9 ug/kg) a similar reduction in intraoperative hypertension was found with the new opioid.[41] In addition, speed of induction was faster with sufentanil.

Inhalation Anesthesia

While speed of anesthetic induction is necessarily slower with inhalation anesthetics used without supplements, an appropriate ultra-short acting intravenous induction agent employed shortly before or after patients are breathing halothane, isoflurane or enflurane makes this type of induction as fast as any other. The real potential problem with induction of anesthesia with inhalation anesthetics is the lack of profound analgesia during endotracheal intubation and the resulting tachycardia and hypertension. This can be overcome by insuring that patients are well anesthetized (have sufficient concentrations of the inhalation agent on board to produce tracheal analgesia). However, adequate concentrations of inhalation anesthesia require time. But is an anesthetic induction which takes 5-10 minutes minutes, instead of 1-2, really that slow, especially if the result is greater hemodynamic stability?

Alternatively, induction of anesthesia with inhalation anesthetics can be very rapid with little risk of hemodynamic instability prior to and following endotracheal intubation, by employing 5-10 ug/kg of fentanyl followed by sodium thiopental (1-1.5 mg/kg) or etomidate (0.1-0.2 mg/kg) while the patient is breathing a tolerable concentration of halothane, enflurane or isoflurane. After paralysis with succinylcholine or an appropriate non-depolarizing muscle relaxant and endotracheal intubation, the inhalation anesthetic concentration is adjusted to maintain arterial blood pressures at desired levels. A slightly different technique which is especially useful in patients with coronary artery disease undergoing coronary artery bypass grafting is the use of high doses of fentanyl (25-40 ug/kg) plus oxygen for anesthetic induction and intubation followed by appropriate concentrations of the inhalation anesthetic. Advantages of this approach are a rapid, hemodynamically event-free anesthetic induction, less possibility of cardiovascular depression (which will occasionally occur with thiopental or etomidate when they are given with or shortly after fentanyl) and less need for high concentrations of the potent inhalation agent during the maintenance phase of the anesthetic.

Induction with inhalation agents without supplements can be accomplished in patients with cardiac disease equally easily with isoflurane, enflurane or halothane. Recent studies suggest that if isoflurane is the agent of choice that induction is most rationally conducted by allowing patients to spontaneously ventilate for the first few moments, and then gradually taking over ventilation so that it becomes controlled shortly thereafter. The reason for this is that patients subjected to controlled ventilation are less likely to experience increases in arterial PaCO.[45] As a result, cardiac output will remain unchanged, arterial blood pressure will decrease slightly (because of a decrease in peripheral resistance) and heart rate will only increase a small amount. When patients are allowed to breathe spontaneously and thus have elevated $PaCO_2$ (because of isoflurane induced respiratory depression), the cardiovascular response to isoflurane is somewhat different. In these patients heart rate and cardiac output are markedly increased.[45] These respiratory changes appear to be much more significant with isoflurane than halothane or enflurane.

Muscle Relaxants

Muscle relaxants are used for facilitating tracheal intubation, providing intercostal muscle paralysis so that sternal spread is less traumatic, preventing movements during light levels of anesthesia, eliminating diaphragmatic muscle movements and allowing controlled mechanical ventilation. Although atracurium and vecuronium, the new short acting non-depolarizing muscle relaxants are available and are undoubtedly changing the practice of anesthesiologists, the most common muscle relaxants up until recently were pancuronium, d-tubocurarine, dimethyltubocurarine, and succinylcholine. The most popular of these agents used for endotracheal intubation have been succinylcholine and pancuronium while d-tubocurarine, dimethyltubocurarine and pancuronium all were frequently employed during maintenance of anesthesia.

The rational use of modern anesthetics dictates that muscle relaxants also be employed with forethought and care. Since all of these agents can produce cardiovascular changes, their selection for use in specific patients should be dictated by that patient's previous medication history, specific premedication, and planned anesthetic drug sequence during both induction and maintenance. It makes little sense to employ agents or use techniques that multiply the chance for detrimental changes in hemodynamics. An example of this would be a patient having anesthesia induced with sodium thiopental, being paralyzed with a large dose of pancuronium for endotracheal intubation and having isoflurane as the maintenance anesthetic. Each of these agents is capable of increasing heart rate and pancuronium when administered as a large bolus dose may also increase arterial blood pressure,[46] particularly after a rapid sequence induction with sodium thiopental without use of an analgesic (Stanley TH, unpublished data).

In patients with CAD the use of a large dose of pancuronium for endotracheal intubation is rarely indicated (in this author's opinion) because of the possibility of tachycardia and hypertension. A possible exception might be the patient receiving large doses of beta-blocking drugs preoperatively and subjected to a high dose narcotic induction sequence. The latter technique can result in significant bradycardia[7,47] and some clinicians reason that use of a large dose of pancuronium is effective in preventing this change.[28,48] Unfortunately, a large dose of pancuronium may overwhelm any narcotic induced bradycardia and result in tachycardia.[7,28,46] For this reason when employing narcotics for anesthetic induction, before use of inhalation maintenance anesthesia, we use a belladonna premedication (to prevent bradycardia) and employ succinylcholine for endotracheal intubation.[47] Similarly, the use of large (bolus) doses of pancuronium following endotracheal intubation is also irrational, for similar reasons, especially in patients having isoflurane for maintenance anesthesia. Rather, a more rational approach, at least from the cardiovascular point of view, would be to administer the drug in small (1-2 mg) increments until the desired level of muscle relaxation is achieved.

Following endotracheal intubation during maintenance inhalation anesthesia with halothane, enflurane or isoflurane, a large bolus of pancuronium may be quite desirable in patients who, for whatever reason, tend to have lower than desirable heart rates and arterial blood pressures and should be used in this situation. On the other hand, a much more rational approach in a patient with hypertension, tachycardia and an elevated cardiac output would be a large dose of d-tubocurarine (30 mg, perhaps given in divided doses) dimethyltubocurarine or the newer, shorter relaxants, atracurium and vecuronium. Even in patients with acceptable hemodynamics, use of the curare-like drugs may be more advantageous than a sympathomemetic like pancuronium, if for example, hemodynamics are on the high side of normal and a particularly stressful surgical stimulus is soon to occur.

Pancuronium and succinylcholine, as well as gallamine (a neuromuscular blocking agent not frequently used in patients with cardiac problems), result in more profound neuromuscular blockade in humans anesthetized with isoflurane than an equi-potent dose of halothane or nitrous oxide plus narcotic compounds.[49,50] For example, the median effective dose of pancuronium necessary to produce 50 percent depression of twitch height was 0.27 mg/m^2 during isoflurane anesthesia and 0.49 mg/m^2 during halothane anesthesia.[51] Similarly, curare is more potent in the presence of isoflurane than halothane.[52]

Maintenance of Anesthesia

It is clear that whether or not they are used during induction of anesthesia, inhalation anesthetics are frequently used in patients undergoing cardiac operations during maintenance phases of anesthetic technique.[46,53,54] Although it is impossible to exactly determine which of the inhalation agents available is most popular, it appears that all are used and that while some clinicians use them without supplementation, most add narcotics and a multiplicity of other agents to reduce inhalation requirements to help optimize myocardial and peripheral vascular hemodynamics.[46,54] Some clinicians feel strongly that mixing opioids and other supplements with inhalation agents is the most rational approach to patients with or without cardiac disease. They cite that opioids and beta blockers can result in easier control of heart rate.[55,56] They add that selective use of nitrates, beta blockers, calcium blockers, nitroglycerin, alpha-adrenergic agonists and similar compounds are most effective in optimizing arterial blood pressure, myocardial contractility, left and right ventricular pre- and afterload, pulmonary and systemic vascular resistances and cardiac output and, therefore, are the best way of providing the ideal depth of anesthesia and protection to the heart.[55,56] Furthermore, they advocate that with one or more of the above titration of the inhalation agent "to effect" is extremely easy and, therefore, that recovery can be rapid, if that is desirable (early extubation) or slower (more opioid--later extubation). These are valid comments and taken in the broadest sense very desirable. However, one problem with this approach is that it leads to maximal polypharmacy and the potential for many drug interactions.

This author tends to be much more of a pharmacologic purist. Thus, when I mix opioids and inhalation agents, I try to avoid the use of other cardiovascularly acting drugs if at all possible. This can be done by increasing the dose of the opioid (usually fentanyl) and/or changing the concentration of the inhalation agent (usually isoflurane) to create the ideal pharmacological and physiological "atmosphere." Consequently, if systemic vascular resistance is a problem, blood pressure is adequate and the patient sufficiently anesthetized, the logical choice is a higher concentration of isofurane which is an ideal "inhalation vasodilator" even in low concentrations and during cardopulmonary bypass. Usually the result is that cardiac output (or flow) remains unchanged and resistance is rapidly decreased without the risk of "over shoot" so common with many of the intravenous vasodilators. While it is not always possible to simply use opioids and inhalation anesthetics, for example, with severe atrial tachycardia, it often is, and the result is an appropriate effect and an easier to understand pharmacologic picture. It is also important to emphasize that inhalation and intravenous anesthetics may produce serious cardiovascular, respiratory and other organ system problems when mixed with many of the popular supplements, i.e., significant and perhaps prolonged cardiovascular depression when mixed with calcium channel blockers.[57] Therefore, in this author's opinion the simplest, most drug free technique that gets the job done is the best.

Conclusion

The skill of the anesthesiologist or his technique as well as his or her understanding of the pathology, the operation, and specific pharmacology and physiology are more important than the choice of any specific anesthetic agent.

References

1. Lowenstein E, Hallowell P, Levine FH, Daggett WM, Austin G, Laver MB: Cardiovascular response to large doses of intravenous morphine in man. N Engl J Med 281:1389-1393, 1969
2. Lowenstein E: Morphine "anesthesia"--A perspective. Anesthesiology 35:563-565, 1971
3. Stoelting RK, Gibbs PS: Hemodynamic effects of morphine and morphine-nitrous oxide in valvular heart disease and coronary artery disease. Anesthesiology 38:45-52, 1973
4. Stanley TH, Gray NH, Stanford W, Armstrong R: The effects of high-dose morphine on fluid and blood requirements in open-heart procedures. Anesthesiology 38:536-541, 1973
5. Hasbrouk JD: Morphine anesthesia for open heart surgery. Ann Thorac Surg 10:364-369, 1970
6. Arens JF, Benbow BP, Ochsner JL, Theard R: Morphine anesthesia for aorto-coronary bypass procedures. Anesth Analg 51:901-909, 1972
7. Stanley TH: The pharmacology of intravenous narcotic anesthetics, Anesthesia. Edited by Miller RD. New York, Churchill Livingstone, 1981, pp 425-449
8. Philbin DM, Moss J, Akins CW, Rosow CE, Kono K, Schneider RC, Verlee TR, Savarese JJ: The use of H_1 and H_2 histamine agonists with morphine anesthesia: A double-blind study. Anesthesiology 55:212-217, 1981
9. Stoelting RK: Influence of barbiturate anesthetic induction on circulatory responses to morphine. Anesth Analg 56:615-617, 1977
10. Stoelting RK, Creasser CE, Gibbs PS: Circulatory effects of halothane added to morphine anesthesia in patients with coronary artery disease. Anesth Analg 53:449-445, 1974

11. Stanley TH: The rational use of inhalation anesthetics during coronary artery surgery, Anesthesia for Cardiovascular Surgery. Edited by Stanley TH, Petty C. Martinus Nijhoff BV, The Hague, 1984, pp 72-83

12. Stanley TH, Webster LR: Anesthetic requirements and cardiovascular effects of fentanyl-oxygen and fentanyl-diazepam-oxygen anesthesia in man. Anesth Analg 57:411-416, 1978

13. Lunn JK, Webster LR, Stanley TH, Woodward A: High dose fentanyl anesthesia for coronary artery surgery: Plasma fentanyl concentration and influence of nitorus oxide on cardiovascular responses. Anesth Analg 58:390-395, 1979

14. Lappas DG, Fahmy NR, Moss J, Salter EE: Effects of fentanyl-diazepam anesthesia on hemodynamics, plasma catecholamines and renin activity in critically ill patients. Anesthesiology 55:A250, 1981

15. Tomichek RC, Rosow CE, Schneider RC, Moss J, Philbin DM; Cardiovascular effects of diazepam-fentanyl anesthesia in patients with coronary artery disease. Anesth Analg 61:271-218, 1982

16. Bailey PL, Pace NL, Stanley TH: Rigidity and hemodynamics during fentanyl induction: Pretreatment with diazepam and pancuronium. Anesthesiology 59:A316, 1983

17. Stanley TH, Berman L, Green O, Robertson D: Plasma catecholamine and cortisol responses to fentanyl-oxygen anesthesia for coronary artery operations. Anesthesiology 53:250-253, 1980

18. Comstock MK, Carter JG, Moyers JR, Stevens WC: Ridigidy and hypercarbia associated with high dose fentanyl induction of anesthesia. Anesth Analg 60:362-363, 1981

19. Coe V, Shafer A, White PF: Technique for administering alfentanil during outpatient anesthesia--a comparison with fentanyl. Anesthesiology 59:A347, 1983

20. Jaffe TB, Ramsey FM: Attenuation of fentanyl-induced truncal rigidity. Anesthesiology 58:562-564, 1983

21. Christian CM, Waller JL, Moldenhauer CC: Postoperative rigidity following fentanyl anesthesia. Anesthesiology 58:265-277, 1983

22. de Lange S, Stanley TH, Boscoe M: Fentanyl-oxygen anesthesia: Comparison of anesthetic requirements and cardiovascular responses in Salt Lake City and Leiden, Holland. Proceedings of the Seventh World Congress of Anaesthesiology. Edited by Zindler M, Rugheimer E. Amsterdam, Excerpta Medica, 1980, p 313

23. Stoelting RK, Gibbs PS, Creasser CW, Peterson C: Hemodynamic and ventilatory responses to fentanyl, fentanyl-droperidol, and nitrous oxide in patients with acquired valvular heart disease. Anesthesiology 42:319-324, 1975

24. Wong WC: Narcotics are not expected to produce unconsciousness and amnesia. Anesth Analg 62:625-626, 1983

25. Stanley TH: High dose narcotic anesthesia. Semin Anesth 1:21-32, 1982

26. Stanley TH: Narcotics as complete anesthetics, Trends in Intravenous Anesthesia. Edited by Aldrete JA, Stanley TH. Chicago, Year Book Medical Publishers, 1980, pp 367-384

27. Lowenstein E, Philbin DM: Narcotic "anesthesia" in the eighties. Anesthesiology 55:195-197, 1981

28. Sebel PS, Bovell JG, Boekhorst RAA, Rog P: Cardiovascular effects of high dose fentanyl anaesthesia. Acta Anesthesiol Scand 26:308-315,

29. Bovill JG, Sebel PS: Pharmacokinetics in high-dose fentanyl: A study in patients undergoing cardiac surgery. Br J Anaesth 52:795-801, 1980

30. Quinton L, Whalley DG, Wynands JE, Morin JE, Mayer R: Oxygen-high dose fentanyl-droperidol anesthesia for aorto-coronary bypass surgery. Anesth Analg 60:412-426, 1981

31. Wynands JE, Townsend GE, Wong P, Whalley DG, Cormbatore BS, Patel YC: Blood pressure response and plasma fentanyl concentration during high and very high dose fentanyl anesthesia for coronary artery surgery. Anesth Analg 62:661-665, 1983

32. Hill AB, Nahrwold ML, de Rosayro M, Knight PR, Jones RM, Bolles RE: Prevention of rigidity during fentanyl-oxygen induction of anesthesia. Anesthesiology 55:452-454, 1981

33. Sebel PS, Bovill JG, Wauquier A, Rog P: Effects of high dose fentanyl anesthesia on the electroencephalogram. Anesthesiology 55:203-211, 1981

34. Mark JB, Greenberg LM: Intraoperative awareness and hypertensive crisis during high dose fentanyl-diazepam anesthesia. Anes Analg 62:698-700, 1983

35. Hilgenberg JC: Intraoperative awareness during high-dose fentanyl oxygen anesthesia. Anesthesiology 54:341-343, 1981

36. Mummaneni N, Rao TLK, Montoya A: Awareness and recall with high-dose fentanyl-oxygen anesthesia. Anesh Analg 59:948-949, 1980

37. Kentor ML, Schwalk AJ, Lieberman RW: Rapid high-dose fentanyl induction for CABG. Anesthesiology 53:S95, 1980

38. Schleimer R, Benjamini E, Eisele J: Pharmacokinetics of fentanyl as determined by radioimmunoassay. Clin Pharmacol Ther 23:188-194, 1978

39. McClain DA, Hug CC: Intravenous fentanyl kinetics. Clin Pharmacol Ther 28: 106-114, 1980

40. Hess R, Stiebler G. Herz A: Pharmacokinetics of fentanyl in man and rabbit. Eur J Clin Pharmacol 4:137-141, 1972

41. de Lange S, Stanley TH, Boscoe M, Pace N: Comparison of sufentanil-O_2 and fentanyl-O_2 anesthesia in man. Anesthesiology 56:112-118, 1982

42. Howie MB, Rietz J, Reilley TE, Harrrington K, Smith D, Dasta JF: Does sufentanil's shorter half-life have any clinical significance? Anesthesiology 59:A146, 1983

43. Reddy P, Liu WS, Port D, Gillmor S, Stanley TH: Comparison of haemodynamic effects of anaesthetic doses of alphaprodine and sufentanil in the dog. Can Anaesth Soc J 27:345-350, 1980

44. Sebel PS, Bovill JG: Cardiovascular effects of sufentanil anesthesia: A study in patients undergoing cardiac surgery. Anesth Analg 61:115-119, 1982

45. Cromwell TH, Stevens WC, Eger EI II, et al: The cardiovascular effects of compound 469 (Forane) during spontaneous ventilation and CO_2 challenge in man. Anesthesiology 35:17-25, 1971

46. Waller JL, Hug CC Jr, Nagle DM et al: Hemodynamic changes during fentanyl-oxygen anesthesia for aorto-coronary bypass operation. Anesthesiology 55:212-217, 1981

47. Stanley TH, Philbin DM, Coggins CH. Fentanyl-oxygen anesthesia for coronary artery surgery: Cardiovascular and anti-diuretic hormone responses. Can Anaesth Soc J 26:168-172, 1979

48. Wynands JE, Wong P, Whalley DG et al: Oxygen fentanyl anesthesia and plasma fentanyl concentations in patients with poor left ventricular function. Anesth Analg 62:476-482, 1983

49. Ali HH, Savarese JJ: Monitoring of neuromuscular function. Anesthesiology 45:216-249, 1976

50. Stevens WC, Cromwell TH, Halsey MJ et al: The cardiovascular effects of a new inhalation anesthetic, Forane, in human volunteers at constant arterial carbon dioxide tension. Anesthesiology 35:8-16, 1971

51. Miller RD, Way WL, Dolan WM, et al: Comparative neuromuscular effects of pancuronium, gallamine and succinylcholine during Forane and halothane anesthesia in man. Anesthesiology 35:509-514, 1971

52. Miller RD, Eger EI II, Way WL et al: Comparative neuromuscular effects of Forane and halothane alone and in combination with d-turbocurarine in man. Anesthesiology 35:38-42, 1971

53. Wynands JE, Townsend GE, Ping Wong BS, et al: Blood pressure response and plasma fentanyl concentrations during high and very high dose fentanyl anesthesia for coronary artery surgery. Anesth Analg 62:661-665, 1983

54. Delaney TJ, Kistner JR, Lake CL etr al: Myocrdial function during halothane and enflurane anesthesia in patients with coronary arery disease. Anesth Analg 59:240-244, 1980

55. Waller JL, Kaplan JA, Jones EL: Anesthesia for coronary revascularization. In: Cardiac Anesthesia, Clinical Cardiology Monographs. Kaplan JA (ed.). Grune and Stratton, New York , 1979, pp 241-280

56. Thomas SJ: Anesthesia considerations for cornoary revascularization. In ASA Refresher Course Lectures, Oct. 1982, p 201

57. Reves JG: Calcium channel blockers and anesthesia. In New Anesthetic Agents, Devices and Monitoring Techniques, edited by Stanley TH and Petty WC, Martin Nijhoff, The Hague, 1983, pp 67-76

DETECTION OF MYOCARDIAL ISCHEMIA DURING ANESTHESIA

S. REIZ, S. HAGGMARK, G. JOHANSSON, M. OSTMAN, E. LOWENSTEIN

INTRODUCTION

Depression, elevation or pseudo-normalization of the electrocardiographic ST-T-segment, are by far the most accepted indicators of myocardial ischemia during anesthesia.Classically, a change of 0.1 mV, measured 80 ms after the maximal R-wave, is the minimal criterion to establish the diagnosis (1). If the electrocardiogram (ECG) is not recorded on paper such small changes are likely to pass undetected. When the different electrocardiographic leads were compared in association with exercise testing, it was found that approximately 90% of all changes suggesting subendocardial ischemia were seen in the V5 lead (2). This lead reflects metabolic changes occurring in the area of the myocardium perfused by the left anterior (LAD) and circumflex (CX) arteries (3). During anesthesia, ischemia in this part of the myocardium is also likely to result in the most severe cardiovascular dysfunction and the highest incidence of early postoperative reinfarction and deaths (4). Monitoring of the V5 lead has consequently been recommended as the minimal requirement for patients with cardiovascular disease, subjected to anesthesia and surgery (5). The use of microprocessor operated oscilloscopes, which graphically present a summary of the ST-T-segments from a multiple lead ECG, have recently been reported to improve the diagnosis of myocardial ischemia (6). As yet, there are however no studies performed in anesthetized patients reporting on the relationship between ECG changes and metabolic changes occurring in the monitored area of the myocardium.

In experimental ischemia it has been shown that mechanical dysfunction occurs before ECG changes are observed (7). This has led to development of new monitoring techniques for detection of myocardial ischemia such as the trans-esophageal, two dimensional echocardiographic technique (2-D echo) recording wall motion abnormality, the nuclear stethoscope, by which ejection fraction can be determined and the cardiokymograph (CKG) which records anterior wall motion. All these techniques have been shown to have considerably greater sensitivity than the ECG in detecting myocardial ischemia (8, 9, 10).

The aim of this presentation is to report on the magnitude of metabolic changes in the area of the myocardium perfused by the LAD required to produce ischemic ST-T-changes in the ECG V5 lead. Furthermore, the ability of the V5 lead and the CKG to detect such metabolic changes is determined and discussed.

MATERIALS

Study I

Fourteen patients without a history of angina pectoris or myocardial infarction formed the control group. They all had a normal electrocardiogram at rest and during exercise, a normal 2-D echo and did not take any medication. These patients were compared to 13 individuals with angina pectoris and/or previous myocardial infarction (q-waves on ECG), positive exercise test or, if the latter could no be conducted, a 2-D echo showing a- or dyskinetic left ventricular wall motion. The patients in the control group were all subjected to major abdominal surgical procedures, whereas all patients with ischemic heart disease were to undergo reconstruction of the abdominal aorta or the common iliac arteries. In the ischemic heart disease group, only patients who demonstrated both periods of an electrocardiogram comparable to the preanesthetic one and periods with depression or elevation of the ST-T-segment of 0.1 mV or more 80 ms after the maximal R-wave, were included.

Study II

In this study, 20 patients with ischemic heart disease, defined as in study I were investigated. No patient with an abnormal preoperative CKG was included. They were all scheduled for major vascular reconstructive surgery on the abdominal aorta or the common iliac arteries.

All patients participated in the two studies after their informed consent had been obtained and the studies were approved by the Ethics Committee of the University of Umea.

METHODS

Patients were premedicated with meperidine, 1-1.5 mg/kg im. Patients without ischemic heart disease had an arterial catheter inserted into the radial artery and a coronary sinus catheter introduced into the great cardiac vein under fluoroscopy. The insertions were made under local anesthesia in the operating room. Patients with ischemic heart disease had the same type of catheters placed and, in addition, a flow directed pulmonary artery thermodilution catheter, wedging in the right lower lobe pulmonary artery.

In study II, the CKG was placed over the anterior wall by te aid of fluoroscopy.

After a 20 min resting period, baseline measurements were performed and the patients were then anesthetized with 4-6 mg/kg of iv thiopentone. Intubation was performed after suxamethonium 1.5 mg/kg and muscle relaxation was maintained with pancuronium bromide 0.1 mg/kg and incremental doses of 1 mg for each half hour following the first hour of anesthesia. Ventilation was controlled by an Engström ECS 2000 volume cycled ventilator and end-tidal carbon dioxide tension maintained around 4.2 kPa. Anesthesia, in all patients, was maintained with isoflurane-nitrous oxide/oxygen (70/30).

In the control group, simultaneous blood samples for lactate analysis (11) were drawn from the artery and the great cardiac vein before anesthesia, 2-3 min after endotracheal intubation, during steady state anesthesia and 10 min after commencement of surgery. The catheters were then removed. In patients with ischemic heart desease, blood samples were drawn as in the control group and in addition, 30 min after commencement of surgery. The coronary sinus catheter was removed at the end of surgery. Only the CKG-s which were accepted by two independent readers were included. All methods have been described in detail elsewhere (12, 13).

The Wilcoxon and Mann-Whitney tests and conventional regression analysis were used for the statistical analyses of the results, which are presented as means $\pm$ SEM. A p-value less than 0.05 was considered statistically significant.

RESULTS

Study I

In the control group there was no change in myocardial lactate extraction from before anesthesia to steady state anesthesia or surgery, nor were any ECG changes recorded. One of 35 (3%) observations demonstrated a greater than 50% reduction in myocardial lactate extraction. Lactate production was not observed (fig. 1).

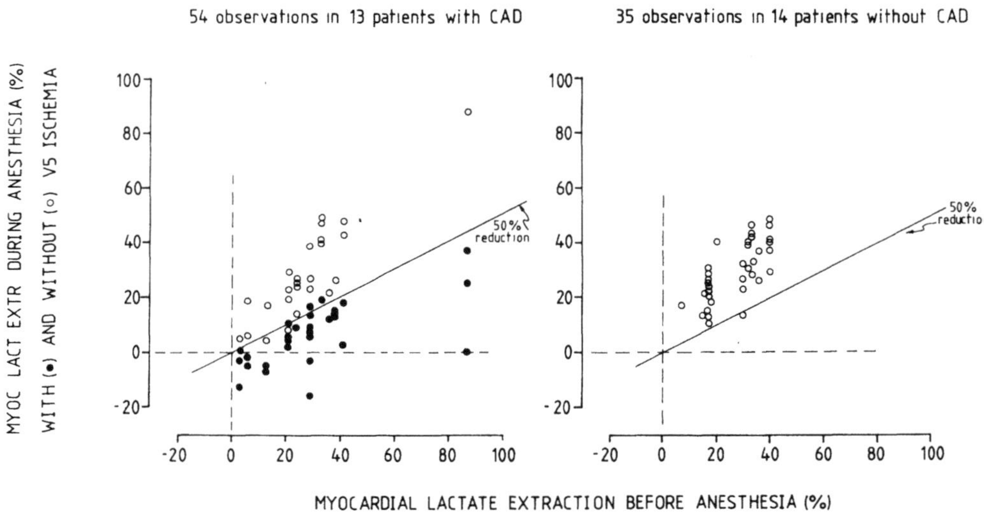

Fig. 1. Myocardial lactate extraction in the area drained by the great cardiac vein of patients with (left) and without (right) coronary artery disease. Note that the 50% reduction line discrimates well between ischemic (closed symbols) and non-ischemic (open symbols) ECG episodes.

In the patients with ischemic heart disease, the periods with new ECG abnormality were associated with a reduction in myocardial lactate extraction by an average $96 \pm 7\%$ ($p<0.001$) compared with the pre/anesthetic value and the control group. There were 9 observations with lactate production. Periods with unchanged ECG were not associated with any change in lactate extraction and did not differ from the control group. The 50% reduction line for lactate extraction discriminated 93% of the ischemic and 92% of the non-ischemic ECG episodes (fig. 1).

Study II

The metabolic goal standard to test the sensitivity of the V5 ECG lead and the CKG were set to a 50% or greater reduction in myocardial lactate extraction in the area perfused by the LAD and drained by the great cardiac vein.

The V5 ECG was found to have a sensitivity of 57% and a specificity of

94% in detecting these changes. The corresponding values for the CKG were 90% and 88% respectiverly. 6.5% of the CKG-s were discarded due to different interpretations by the two independent readers. With concordant ECG and CKG, the sensitivity was 93% and the specificity was 96%. 8 of 10 periods with lactate production were detected by the CKG compared with 5 of 10 by the ECG (fig. 2).

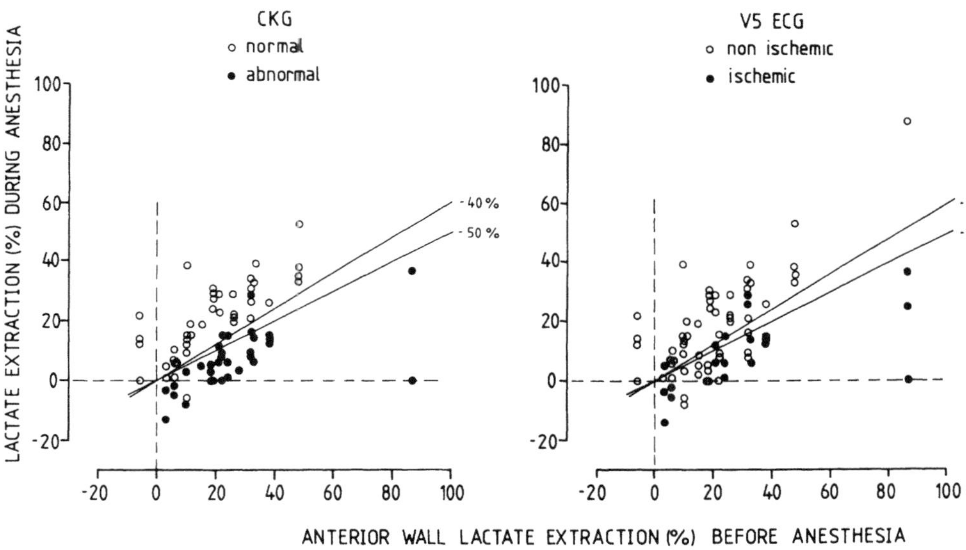

Fig. 2. Abnormal (closed symbols) and normal (open symbols ECG and CKG episodes in relation to myocardial lactate extraction in the area drained by the great cardiac vein of patients with coronary artery disease. Note, that the ECG only detects half the periods with lactate production (right panel).

DISCUSSION

The incidence of myocaridal ischemia during anesthesia and surgery in patients with ischemic heart disease subjected to non-cardiac surgery is high (14). Using one of the three criteria, ST-T-segment changes, abnormal wall motion or myocardial lactate production, we have found that 50-60% of patients with coronary artery disease become ischemic during one or more periods of anesthesia and surgery regardless of the anesthetic agent chosen. The mechanisms for development of ischemia may

however vary with the anesthetic agent chosen, its dose and the magnitude of surgical stimulation.
The different methods of detecting ischemia do not follow the same time course. Furthermore they all have limitations, mostly related to how selectively they monitor the area at risk.

ANALYSIS OF MYOCARDIAL LACTATE METABOLISM

Lactate is used as a substrate by the myocardium. In ischemia, lactate is produced and may, provided the ischemic area is large enough, offset a negative concentration gradient between arterial and coronary venous blood. During undisturbed anesthesia, coronary perfusion pressure is frequently markedly decreased and the flow over a stenosis may be reduced to an extent where the contribution from the area behind the stenosis, to total venous outflow, may be very small. Under such circumstances and in case of ischemia in this area, it is unlikely that myocardial lactate extraction is more than marginally decreased. During intubation and surgical stress, the circulation may be hyperdynamic, resulting in increased flow to non-constricted areas and insufficient flow to poststenotic areas. Consequently, lactate from ischemic areas may be diluted and offset a minor fall in lactate extraction only. Part, but not the whole of the problem may be solved by more selective coronary venous sampling. For this purpose we chose to catheterize the great cardiac vein to study the lactate metabolism in the area of the myocardium perfused by the LAD.
Patients in whom we could not find any evidence of coronary artery disease, did not show any change in myocardial lactate extraction during anesthesia and surgery. There was no correlation between arterial lactate concentration and myocardial lactate extraction, as previously reported in healthy volunteers subjected so successive elevation of heart rate by atrial pacing (15). The authors of this study concluded that a low positive lactate extraction value (below 10%, which was seen in 20% of their patients) would not necessarily indicate ischemia. They also recommend that only lactate production should be used as evidence of ischemia.
In the patient group with coronary artery disease, we had selected to study only those who presented both an ECG comparable to the preanesthetic one and an ischemic ECG during induction, undisturbed

anesthesia and/or surgery. In this group, we found that myocardial lactate extraction during or after induction of anesthesia or during surgery was not different from the awake mean value as long as the ECG had not changed and, also not different from the mean value measured in patients without coronary artery disease under the same conditions. In contrast to the control group and to the non-ischemic ECG periods, there was a highly significant fall in lactate extraction ($96 \pm 7\%$, $p<0.001$), when ECG abnormality was first observed (fig.1). A total of nine episodes of lactate production, all with abnormal ECG, were observed. A 50% reduction in myocardial lactate extraction was associated with development of ST-T-changes of 0.1 mV or more in 93% of the instances. Similarly, 92% of unchanged ECG-s were associated with a less than 50% reduction in myocardial lactate extraction. Like in the control group, there was no correlation between arterial lactate concentration and myocardial lactate extraction in the patients with coronary artery disease.

Based on our observations, we agree with Gertz et al (15) that a single low, positive myocardial lactate extraction value is not diagnostic for regional myocardial ischemia. However, if myocardial lactate extraction falls by more than 50% from the awake control value with induction of anesthesia and commencement of surgery, one should suspect regional myocardial ichemia. As long as lactate production is not present one should however not rely solely on the metabolic criterion but use complementary methods to finally establish the diagnosis.

ANALYSIS OF THE V5 ECG AND THE CKG TO DETECT METABOLIC CHANGES IN THE ANTERIOR MYOCARDIAL WALL

We studied the V5 lead because this is the most commonly used lead and has been reported to detect around 90% of all electrocardiographically demonstrable ischemic events. However, the V3 and V4 leads more adequately monitor the area perfused by the LAD.

When comparing the ability of the V5 ECG and the CKG to detect a fall in myocardial lactate extraction of 50% or greater as determined from sampling in the great cardiac vein, we found the CKG to have a far greater sensitivity (90% versus 57%). The same relationship between the sensitivity of the two methods was found, when lactate production only was used as the goal standard for ischemia. When both ECG and CKG became abnormal, the ECG abnormality always occurred after the CKG abnormality and stayed abnormal for a shorter period than the CKG. The CKG could remain abnormal for several hours after normalization of the ECG. The ECG had a better sensitivity than the CKG (96% versus 88%). This difference was due to a few abnormal CKG-s developing in association with surgically induced hypertension. This happened in patients with akinesia in part of the anterior wall as detected by the preoperative 2-D echo. We suggest that the CKG abnormality, in these patients, was due to pure mechanical dysfunction, following increase in impedance to left ventricular ejection rather than to ischemia.

In conclusion, we found the CKG to be a sensitive monitor of metabolic changes in the anterior myocardial wall suggesting ischemia. In this respect, the CKG was superior to the V5 ECG.

REFERENCES

1. McHenry PL, Fisch C: Clinical applications of the treadmill exercise test. Mod Conc Cardiovasc Dis 46, 46, 21-25, 1977.
2. Blackburn H, Katigbak R: What electrocardiographic leads to take after exercise? Am Heart J 67, 184-186, 1964.
3. Gensini GG, Di Giorgi S, Coskun O, et al: Anatomy of the coronary circulation in living man. Circulation 31, 778-784, 1965.
4. Steen SA, Tinker JH, Tarhan S: Myocardial reinfarction after anesthesia and surgery. JAMA 239, 2566-2570, 1978.
5. Kotrly KJ, Kotter, GS, Mortara D, Kampine JP: Intraoperative detection of myocardial ischemia with an ST-segment trend monitoring system. Anesth Analg 63, 343-345, 1984.
6. Kaplan JA, King SB: The precordial electrocardiographic lead (V5) in patients who have coronary-artery disease. Anesthesiology 45, 570-574, 1976.
7. Water DD, Da Luz P, Wyatt HL et al: Early changes in regional and global left ventricular function induced by graded reductions in regional coronary perfusion. Am J Cardiol 39, 537-543, 1977.
8. Cahalan MK, Kremer P, Schiller NB, et al: Intraoperative monitoring with two-dimensional transesophageal echocardiography. Anesthesiology 57, A153 (abstract), 1982.
9. Barash PG, Barabadkar S, Giles R, et al: Preservations of global left ventricular function during intubation in patients with ischemic heart disease. Anesthesiology 55, A6 (abstract), 1981.
10. Bellows WH, Bode RH Jr, Levy JH, et al: Noninvasive detection of peri-induction ischemic ventricular dysfunction by cardiokymography in man: preliminary experience. Anesthesiology 60, 155-158, 1984.
11. Soutter WP, Sharp F, Clark DM: Bedside estimation of whole blood lactate. Br J Anaesth 50, 445-450, 1978.
12. Reiz S, Balfors E, Sorensen MB, et al: Isoflurane - a powerful coronary vasodilator in patients with coronary artery disease. Anesthesiology 59, 91-97, 1983.

13. Silverberg RA, Diamond GA, Vas R, et al: Noninvasive diagnosis of coronary artery disease: the cardiokymographic stress test. Circulation 61, 579, 1980.
14. Roy WL, Edelist G, Gilbert B: Myocardial ischemia during non-cardiac surgical procedures in patients with coronary artery disease Aensthesiology 51, 393-397, 1979.
15. Gertz EW, Wisneski JA, Neese R, et al: Myocardial lactate extraction: Multi-determined metabolic function. Circulation 61, 256-261, 1980.

THE MANAGEMENT OF INTRAOPERATIVE MYOCARDIAL ISCHEMIA AND HYPOTENSION

Carl C. Hug, Jr., M.D., Ph.D.

The delicate balance between myocardial oxygen supply and demand in the patient with coronary artery disease can be disturbed by any number of factors (Table 1). The anesthesiologist keeps these factors in mind in preventing detrimental changes in myocardial oxygen balance and in treating myocardial ischemia. Of particular importance is the fact that increases in heart rate and increases in ventricular preload disturb myocardial oxygen balance both by decreasing oxygen supply and by increasing its utilization.

Table 1. Detrimental Changes in Myocardial Oxygen Balance

DECREASED MYOCARDIAL OXYGEN SUPPLY	INCREASED MYOCARDIAL OXYGEN DEMAND
1. Decreased coronary blood flow	1. Tachycardia
a. Tachycardia	2. Increased wall tension
b. Diastolic hypotension	a. Increased preload
c. Increased preload	b. Increased afterload
d. Hypocapnia	3. Increased contractility
e. Coronary spasm	
2. Decreased oxygen delivery	
a. Anemia	
b. Hypoxia	
c. Decreased 2,3-DPG	

Both tachycardia and tachyarrhythmias increase ventricular oxygen utilization and reduce oxygen delivery, especially to the subendocardium, because they reduce diastolic perfusion time. They should be treated promptly (Table 2).

Table 2. TACHYCARDIA

Etiology	Therapy
Reflex tachycardia	
- with ↓BP	Phenylephrine, ↑Intravascular volume
- with ↑BP	Propranolol, ↑Anesthesia
Supraventricular dysrhythmia	Propranolol, Verapamil
	Cardioversion
	Ouabain, Digoxin

Because perfusion of the subendocardium is determined by the difference between mean diastolic blood pressure ($\overline{dBP}$) and left ventricular end-diastolic pressure (LVEDP),

$$\text{Coronary Perfusion Pressure (CPP)} = \overline{dBP} - \text{LVEDP}$$

increases in ventricular preload reduce subendocardial perfusion. At the same time, an increased preload increases oxygen utilization by increasing left ventricular wall tension. Nitroglycerin is particularly effective in reducing preload through its actions on systemic veins to increase their capacitance, thereby reducing the return of blood to the heart. Nitroglycerin may also improve coronary blood flow to ischemic areas; at least it appears not to create an unfavorable steal of blood from ischemic areas. At the same time, nitroglycerin tends to reduce systemic vascular resistance and the impedance to left ventricular ejection, thereby reducing myocardial work and oxygen utilization. Of course, a marked reduction in systemic arterial blood pressure, especially mean diastolic pressure, reduces coronary perfusion pressure. In the case of systemic hypotension, the combination of nitroglycerin and phenylephrine allows the favorable effects of nitroglycerin on preload and coronary vascular resistance to be maintained while phenylephrine increases systemic blood pressure. The drug combination favors increased coronary blood flow by increasing dBP (phenylephrine) and decreasing LVEDP (nitroglycerin).

Hypotension from any cause is likely to reduce coronary perfusion pressure, and it should be treated promptly (Table 3). An intravenous injection of phenylephrine (a pure vasopressor) or ephedrine (a mild inotrope and vasopressor) is often helpful in restoring coronary perfusion until the etiology of the systemic hypotension can be corrected. In the acute situation and especially in the patient with good ventricular function, there may be merit in treating hypotension with a pure vasopressor which tends to increase systemic blood pressure and CPP without stimulating the heart and increasing myocardial oxygen demand. Ultimately, when the cause of hypotension is identified, an inotropic drug may be indicated to improve myocardial function and cardiac output. A pure vasopressor may be deterimental to the heart in the patient with poor ventricular function. In either case, after the acute hypotension is corrected, optimal cardiovascular performance is best achieved by the use of sophisticated (invasive) hemodynamic monitoring.

Table 3. THERAPY OF HYPOTENSION
Legs-up position, IV fluids
Sympathomimetic, Calcium
- vasopressor vs inotrope
Correct abnormal rate & rhythm
(Then optimize cardiac output.)

Excessively high systemic blood pressure is associated with increased left ventricular work and oxygen utilization. When hypertensive episodes are associated with myocardial ischemia they should be treated promptly (Table 4). Ideally, the cause of the hypertension should be corrected, but until it is, drug therapy aimed at controlling the hypertension is beneficial.

Table 4. ACUTE THERAPY OF HYPERTENSION
Etiology!
Nitroprusside, Nitroglycerin, Hydralazine
Trimethaphan
Labetalol, Propranolol
Nifedipine

The management of myocardial ischemia, especially in the perioperative period, can be summarized as follows:

Ischemia associated with tachycardia

- increase analgesia, increase anesthetic depth
- propranolol
- verapamil
- nitroglycerin

Ischemia associated with increased preload (↑ PAWP)

- nitroglycerin
- head-up position
- restrict fluids
- inotrope

Ischemia associated with systemic hypotension

- phenylephrine
- if ↑PAWP, nitroglycerin, inotrope
- if ↓PAWP, legs-up position, ↑intravascular volume

Ischemia associated with systemic hypertension

- increase analgesia, increase anesthetic depth
- vasodilator
- propranolol, labetalol

Of course, it is best to avoid myocardial ischemia, and in the patient with coronary artery disease this is most often accomplished by anesthetic management and intensive care plans aimed at maintaining 1) a satisfactorily low ventricular filling pressure, 2) a slow heart rate, 3) an adequate diastolic blood pressure, and 4) by avoiding systemic hypertension.

General References

Cardiac Anesthesia, Volume 2, Cardiovascular Pharmacology, edited by J. A. Kaplan, Grune & Stratton, New York 1983.

- Curling PE, Kaplan JA: Effects of anesthetics on the coronary circulation, p 123-141
- Kaplan JA: Protection of the ischemic myocardium, p 145-149
- Kaplan JA: Nitrates, p 151-180
- Slogoff S: Beta-adrenergic blockers, p 181-208
- Kates RA, Kaplan JA: Calcium channel blocking drugs, p 209-242
- Merin RG: Myocardial metabolism, p 243-263

Hug CC Jr: Management of hemodynamic instability complicated by hypotension. ASA Refresher Courses in Anesthesiology 13: (in press), 1985. (Published by J.B. Lippincott, Philadelphia, Pennsylvania.)

Specific References

Come PC, Flaherty JT, Baird MG, et al: Reversal by phenylephrine of the beneficial effects of intravenous nitroglycerin in patients with acute myocardial infarction. N Engl J Med 293:1003-1007, 1975.

Borer JS, Redwood DR, Levitt B, et al: Reduction in myocardial ischemia with nitroglycerin or nitroglycerin plus phenylephrine administration during acute myocardial infarction. N Engl J Med 293:1008-1012, 1975.

Metabolic changes and interpretation of blood gas analysis during hypothermia

D. KETTLER and E. TURNER
Zentrum Anästhesiologie der Universität Göttingen, Robert-Koch-Str. 40, D-3400 Göttingen

As H. Swan (19) has entitled a review hypothermia is a lady with a past and some promise for the future. The vast history and literature about the clinical use of hypothermia was reviewed in his article in 1973. Since then not much has been added to our knowledge about hypothermia neither has his list of indications for the possible use of hypothermia been practically evaluated. Thus, the future of hypothermia has not yet begun. Nowadays hypothermia ist mainly used in cardiac surgery during cardio-pulmonary bypass and to some extent in neurosurgery for operations on vessel-rich intracranial leasons. These indications are more than 20 years old. Therefore, anesthesiologists who work in cardiac surgery seem to take induced hypothermia as a natural and uncomplicated procedure. But it seems worthwhile to remember the problems which may be associated with hypothermic metabolism, oxygen demand and supply and interpretation of acid base and blood gas analysis if considering possible benefits of hypothermia for other indications. This article will review the well known aspects of hypothermia and outline some possibilities of future research.

1. Metabolic effects of hypothermia

The metabolic effects of hypothermia depend on its own specific action and the regulatory state of the organism which is cooled.

As man is not a poikilothermic or hibernating animal normal body temperature around 36.5 to 37.2°C is defended by effective systems of behavioural and physiological cold defense and heat production.

Metabolism can increase up to sixfold the basal metabolic rate (BMR) when cold is applicated to awake man. Vasoconstriction, increases in cardiac output and blood pressure due to sympathetic stimulation occur during cold stress. This response can be observed down to 27°C in accidental hypothermia (11,22) and is aggravated during rewarming leading to complications because of cardiac arrhythmias or sudden cardiac death. Therefore, the benefits of hypothermia can only be achieved in patients who are anesthetized. This again introduces methodological difficulties when investigating the metabolic effects of hypothermia, because different anesthetics exert different effects on the thermoregulatory response and the resting metabolism.

According to numerous investigations in animals under barbiturate-anesthesia (20) and in man with brain injury (22), during absence of a thermoregulatory response a reduction of whole body oxygen uptake ($\dot{V}O_2$) with hypothermia is observed which has a Q_{10} in the range of 2.5 to 3.0.:

$\log Q_{10} = \frac{10}{T_2 - T_1} \cdot (\log k_2 - \log k_1)$, were T2 and T_1 are the temperatures at which the metabolic rates k_2 and k_1 are measured.

This reduction of metabolic rate is probably the main factor of protection from ischemic damage during hypothermia, because the energy stores become less faster depleted when metabolic demands are low and the cell function is preserved longer. Figure 1 shows the safe time of circulatory arrest and whole body $\dot{V}O_2$ as a function of body temperature.

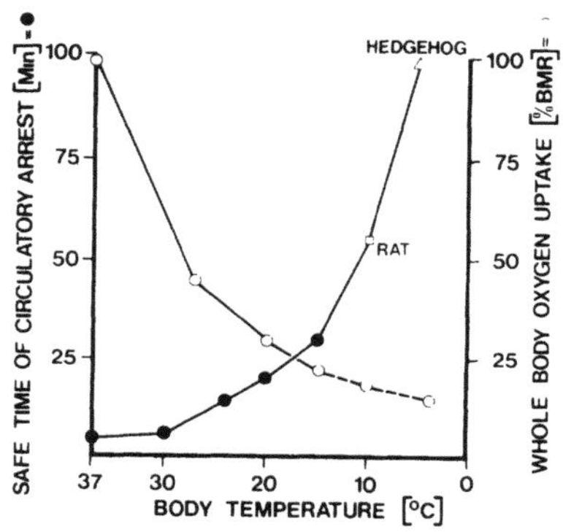

Fig. 1: Safe time of circulatory arrest and whole body oxygen uptake ($\dot{V}O_2$) in relation to body temperature.

At the same rate at which oxygen consumption is decreased during hypothermia an increase in ischemic tolerance time is observed. A functional relationship between the two variables therefore, is highly probable. Prolongation of ischemic tolerance during hypothermia will only be achieved when the thermoregulatory response is suppressed and whole body $\dot{V}O_2$ does not rise. In this context the endocrine metabolic response to cold may be of importance. While anesthesia with the use of muscle-relaxants will prevent shivering it is not sure that the sympathetic response to cold will be suppressed. If not, $\dot{V}O_2$ may increase by 40% during mild hypothermia (7) due to nonshivering thermogenesis. Investigations in man which anesthetic will yield the greatest reduction of $\dot{V}O_2$ during hypothermic cardiopulmonary bypass (CPB) have not been carried out so far and there is no work done in man on the oxygen demands of the brain during hypothermic CPB in relation to different anesthetics. Investigations of Berntmann et.al (1) and Nordström and Rehcrona (16) show that the combination of barbiturates and hypothermia suppresses brain metabolism more than the combination of e.g. nitrous oxide/fentanyl and hypothermia. Therefore barbiturates and hypothermia could yield the greatest possible cerebral protection. Adverse effects of thiopental on cardiac function however, limit its use in cardiac surgery. In our institution we use fentanyl in a combination with flunitrazepam or inhalational anesthetics during CPB to assure that the thermoregulatory response to cold is suppressed and awareness is avoided. Nevertheless we observed a hormonal stress response during CPB (9) when high doses of fentanyl were used. Suppression of the hormonal response by cold itself occurs only below 25°C (14). The estimation of hypothermic organ protection only from the measurement of body temperature may therefore be critical.

Additionally, the relationship of organ protection and body temperature is only applicable for steady state conditions when cooling is not inhomogeneous. These conditions are rare in the clinical situation with rapid cooling, maldistribution of blood flow during onset of CPB and rapid rewarming after short intracardial procedures. Figure 2 shows the temperatures of the different organs during fast bloodstream cooling and rewarming taken from the work done by Peirce et al and published in the book of Galletti and Brecher (5).

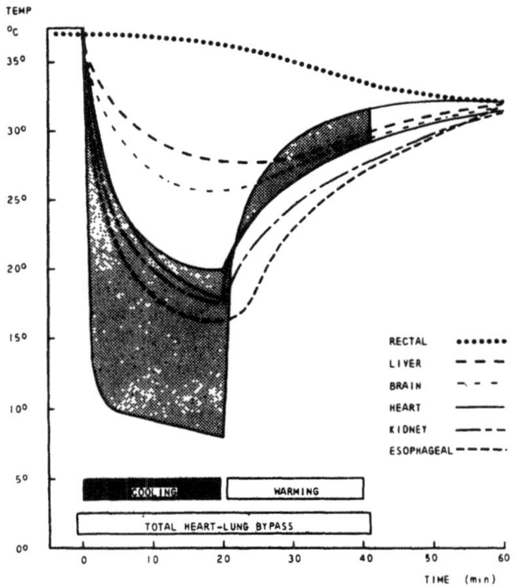

Fig. 2: Temperatures of different organs during fast blood stream cooling in CPB. After Galletti and Brecher (5).

Measuring the rectal and the esophageal temperature will give information about the whole range of temperatures in the body. As you can see brain temperature is nearly in the middle of the two extremes. Esophageal temperature is changing very fast and will therefore lead to overestimation of hypothermic brain protection. The same is true for whole body $\dot{V}O_2$ as is illustrated by figure 3 from the work of Borst (3), who compared surface to blood stream cooling.

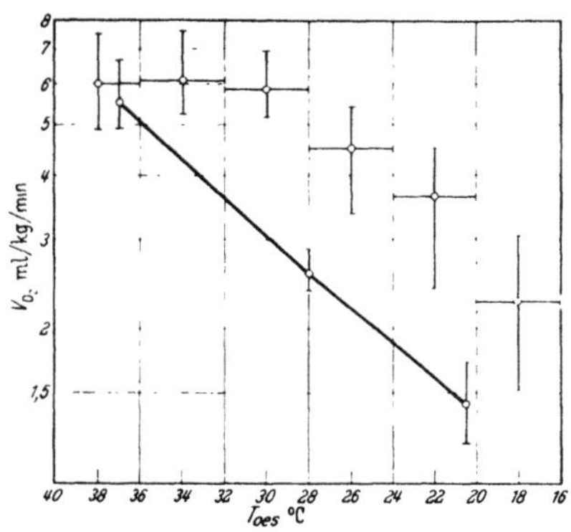

Fig. 3: Oxygen uptake ($\dot{V}O_2$) in relation to esophageal temperature (T_{oes}) during surface cooling (solid line) or blood stream cooling (crosses) from the work of Borst (3).

During blood stream cooling oxygen demand may even rise in the beginning and later drop slowly in relation to esophageal temperature. This is not the case during surface cooling, when esophageal temperature follows the average temperature of the tissues. This phenomenon of inhomogenous cooling must be expected in the clinical situation of hypothermic CPB as well. Homogenous cooling may be enhanced by use of vasodilators when arterial pressure on CPB is high ($\sim$ 100 mmHg). Low blood pressures ($<$ 60mgHg) and low perfusion volumes ($< 2.0\ l \cdot min^{-1} \cdot m^{-2}$) should be avoided before homogenous cold organ protection (rectal temperature about 28°C) is provided.
During rewarming metabolism and oxygen supply are different compared to cooling at equal temperature. Oxygen consumption on CPB rises more during rewarming as may be predicted by the rise in rectal temperature (due to uneven rewarming) but also in relation to esophageal temperature (Figures 4,5). Therefore, it has been often discussed whether either the onset of CPB or the arterial delivery of cold blood decreases oxygen uptake below oxygen demands and induces a limited shock state (21). The accumulated oxygen dept was thought to be repaid during the rewarming period. Lactate decreases as the arterio-mixed venous oxygen content differences are

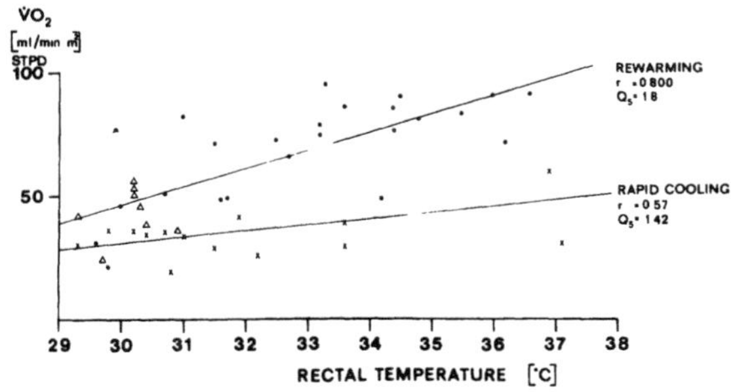

Fig. 4: Whole body oxygen consumption ($\dot{V}O_2$) during cooling and rewarming on CPB in relation to rectal temperature. Own unpublished results.

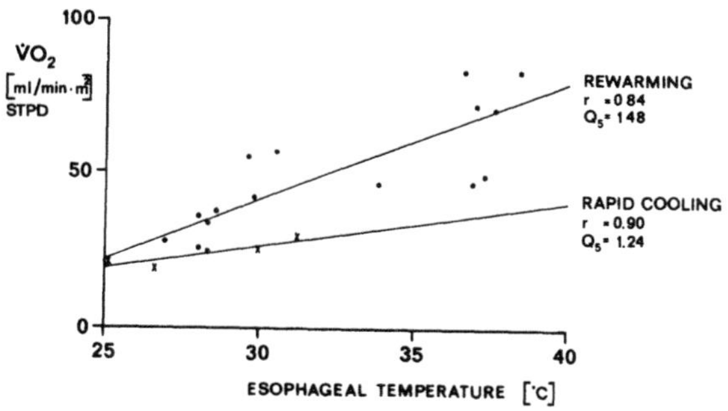

Fig. 5: Whole body oxygen consumption ($\dot{V}O_2$) during cooling and rewarming on CPB in relation to esophageal temperature.
Own unpublished results.

narrow at the beginning of CPB with cooling and wide at the end of CPB. After incomplete rewarming oxygen availability is probably sufficient when high perfusion volumes and modern oxygenators are employed. The initial fall of oxygen uptake may therefore not be representative for the whole period of CPB but include two further factors due to the onset of CPB, namely:
The onset of hypotension and maldistribution of (non pulsatile) blood flow. Because of hemodilution an acute fall in oxygen transport capacity and blood viscosity occurs which with falling temperature (6) is counteracted. These changes may

explain the low $\dot{V}O_2$ during onset of hypothermic CPB. Contradictory in part to this hypothesis are the results of Lundsgaard-Hansen (12) who found a higher exess lactate (XL) during hypothermic than during normothermic CPB. These results would allow the conclusion that the distribution of cold blood leads to some kind of oxygen deficit in contrast to a better distribution of warm blood. Whether this effect is also observed during surface hypothermia is contradictory in the literature (12,20).However, the parameters of oxygen deficit were ambiguous or probably anesthesia not constant in these investigations. For clinical purposes it has to be kept in mind that we are only on the safe side if we do not reduce blood flow during rewarming.
Other metabolic effects of hypothermia include the consequences of endocrine reactions on carbohydrate metabolism. As catecholamines increase during moderate hypothermia and as during surgical procedures the insulin secretion is suppressed a rise in blood glucose is observed (14). Whether cortisol is increased during hypothermia is contradictory (14). During rewarming there is a drop in blood glucose (2) without changes in the level of either catecholamines or free fatty acids. Only corticosteroids seem to decrease during rewarming. Either the decrease of glucocorticoids or a better microcirculation or enzyme function during rewarming could be responsible for the observed drop in blood glucose. High $\dot{V}O_2$ could also be a supporting sign of enhanced metabolism during rewarming. The blood glucose level should therefore be carefully controlled during rewarming because hypoglycemia can occur.

2. Blood gas and acid base changes during hypothermia

At first it has to be considered which in vitro changes occur in blood gas samples drawn from a cold patient which are rewarmed to 37°C in the analyser. The anaerobic changes of whole blood during cooling and heating have been summarized by Severinghaus (18) being transformed into a slide ruler called "blood gas calculator", which is generally used for correction of blood gas analysis for temperature. Today most blood gas analysers have a program for temperature correction. All together the anaerobic changes from temperature yield that a blood gas analysis of a patient at 25°C which is measured at 38°C can be interpreted as "normal" when

$$\text{pH } 38°\text{C} = 7{,}2 \quad — \quad \text{pH } 25°\text{C} = 7{,}4$$

$$pCO_2\ 38°\text{C} = 75 \quad — \quad pCO_2\ 25°\text{C} = 40\ [\text{mmHg}]$$

$$pO_2\ 38°\text{C} > 140 \quad — \quad pO_2\ 25°\text{C} > 55\ [\text{mmHg}]$$

because the solubility of gases in blood increases with falling temperature (partial pressures fall) and the dissociation decreases also with falling temperatures (pH moves to the alkalotic side).
If the actual values of the patient are of importance, temperature correction of blood gas analysis is mandatory.

So far there is general agreement. Problems arise when the

anaesthesiologist has to decide how much ventilation is needed during hypothermia. On cardiopulmonary bypass ventilation within the oxygenator is achieved by high gas flow and high oxygen concentrations because of the limited diffusing capacity for oxygen. As CO_2 diffuses readily through the membrane this leads to an increase in CO_2-removal with severe respiratory alcalosis. Therefore CO_2 has to be added to the gas flow through the oxygenator. The question is how much CO_2 shall be added to the oxygen flow and which PCO_2 and pH values are optimal for a patient during hypothermia.

As the base excess is not influenced during a normothermic high flow (100 ml/kg^{-1}) perfusion with either high (5%) or low (1%) CO_2 concentrations changes in acid base balance due to CPB are nearly completely respiratory (12). The use of buffer substances during CBP therefore is usually not necessary. There are no differences in excess lactate with either high or low CO_2 concentrations during high flow (100 ml·kg^{-1}) CPB (12). Probably the ratio of oxygen supply and demand is not critical during either high or low CO_2 concentrations on hypothermic CPB, although oxygen demand rises with respiratory alkalosis (10, 17, 23). This problem may not be of clinical significance when the oxygen availability is high. On the other hand it may be important to approach a state of the lowest reversible suppression of metabolism and function during ischemic conditions. From investigations on optimal pH and pCO_2 for organ preservation during ischemia (4) we know that keeping pH and pCO_2 during hypothermia in the normothermic range yields the best conditions. In contrast, it is known from other investigations (11, 22) that during accidental hypothermia the best therapeutic results are obtained when the arterial pCO_2 is kept slightly below normal (pCO_2 30-35 mmHg). During accidental hypothermia in most cases this respiratory alkalosis is combined with a metabolic acidosis resulting in a temperature corrected pH of 7.3-7.4. The problem of an optimal pH during hypothermia cannot be solved at this time. It seems wise that extremes in either ventilation or pH should be avoided. Investigations in animals which during hypothermia keep their pH constant at 7.4 (hibernators) or keep the distance to the neutral point of water at 0.6 pH units constant (poikilotherms) are very interesting but are not easily transferable to human biology.

3. Future research

If we want to make hypothermic procedures with or without the use of CPB safe for other indications besides cardiac surgery the following problems have to be solved:

a) Are there significant differences in the mortality after long term hypothermia (e.g. 12 hours) and rewarming of warm blooded animals when either temperature corrected pH and pCO_2 are kept constant or when the relative alkalinity of the body (normal offset 0.6 pH units from the neutral point of water) is maintained? Especially the function of the brain and the heart should be monitored, as keeping the pCO_2 (temperature corrected) constant may be harmful for the heart but desirable for the brain (13).

b) Similar investigations of long term hypothermic CPB should be carried out, where CO_2 effects on the heart may be not so important but on the other hand cerebral edema may develop which would suggest addition of 5% CO_2 during hypothermia to be dangerous (15).

c) Further investigations on the tolerance to hypoxemia during short term hypothermia with either pH constant or constant offset of the pH from neutral point of water could be carried out with the question if a lower oxygen demand during acidosis may be desirable for preservation of organ function during hypoxic conditions or not.

These three examples show how complex the problem of hypothermia as a tool of treatment is. Further experimental work is necessary before the future of induced hypothermia may begin.

REFERENCES

1. Berntmann L., Welsh F.A., Harp J.R. (1981) Cerebral protective effects of low-grade hypothermia. Anesthesiology 55, 495-498
2. Bloch M. (1967) Cerebral effects of rewarming following prolonged hypothermia: Significance for the management of severe cranio cerebral injury and acute pyrexia. Brain 90, 169-784
3. Borst H.G. (1963) Experimentelle Untersuchungen über die kombinierte Anwendung von extrakorporalem Kreislauf und Hypothermie. I. Pathophysiologie der Auskühlung und Wiedererwärmung. Langenbecks Arch. 302, 321-351
4. Bretschneider H.J. (1985) Pers. Kommunikation
5. Galletti P.M., Brecher G.A. (eds) (1962) Heart-Lung Bypass. Principles and Techniques of Extracorporeal Circulation. Grune + Stratton, New York, San Francisco, London, p. 294
6. Gordon R.J., Ravin M., Daicoff G.R. et al. (1973) Effects of hemodilution on hypotension during cardiopulmonary bypass. Anesth. Analg. 54, 482
7. Jessen K. (1980) An assessment of human regulatory nonshivering thermogenesis. Acta Anaesth. Scand. 24, 138-143
8. Hemmingway A. (1963) Shivering. Physiol. Rev. 43, 397-422
9. Kettler D., Hasse F., Hensel, I. (1982) Streßfreie Anästhesie in der Herzchirurgie durch hohe Opiatdosen - gibt es so etwas? In: de Vivie E.R., Hellberg K., Ruschewski W. (eds) Herzchirurgie 1982, TM - Verlag, Bad Oeynhausen, S. 263 - 271
10. Kreienbühl G., Gattiker R. (1976) Der Einfluß der arteriellen Kohlensäurespannung auf den Sauerstoffverbrauch während extrakorporalem Kreislauf in Hypothermie. Anaesthesist 25, 47-50
11. Ledingham I. Mc. A., Mom J.G. (1980) Treatment of accidental hypothermia: A prospective clinical study. Brit. Med. J. 280, 1102
12. Lundsgaard-Hansen P. (1966) Sauerstoffversorgung und Säure-Basenhaushalt in tiefer Hypothermie. Springer, Berlin, New York, Heidelberg (Anästhesiologie und Wiederbelebung Vol. 12)
13. Ohmura A., Wong K.C., Westenskow D.R., Shaw L. (1979) Effects of Hypocarbia and Normocarbia on Cardiovascular Dynamics and Regional Circulation in the Hypothermic Dog. Anesthesiology 50, 293-298
14. Popovic V., Popovic P. (1974) Hypothermia in Biology and in Medicine. Grune + Stratton, New York, San Francisco, London.
15. Ream A.K., Reitz B.A., Silverberg G. (1982) Temperature correction of pCO_2 and ph in Estimating AcidBase Status: An example of the Emperors New Clothes. Anesthesiology 56, 41-44

16. Rehcrona S. (1981) Reduction of cerebral metabolic rate as a possibility for brain protection during carotid endarterectomy. In: Rügheimer E., Zindler M.: Anaesthesiology, Proc. 7th World Congress of Anaesthesiologists, Hamburg, September 14-21, 1980. Excerpta medica, Amsterdam-Oxford-Princeton JCS
17. Schreiner-Heltjen J. (1980) Der Einfluß der arteriellen Kohlensäurespannung und des arteriellen pH-Wertes auf den Sauerstoffverbrauch des Gesamtorganismus während der extracorporalen Zirkulation. Anaesthesist 29, 300-310
18. Severinghaus J.W. (1966) Blood gas calculator. J. Appl. Physiol. 21, 1108-1116
19. Swan H. (1973) Clinical hypothermia: A lady with a past and some promise for the future. Surgery 73, 736-758
20. Thauer R., Brendel W. (1962) Hypothermie. Progr. Surg. 2, 73-271
21. Turner E., Braun U., Leitz K.H., Hilfiker O. (1982) Überwachung der Gesamtsauerstoffaufnahme bei coronarchirurgischen Eingriffen. Anaesthesist 31, 280-286
22. Turner E., Radke J., Hilfiker O., Stafforst D., Braun U., Kettler D.(1984) Wiedererwärmung bei mittlerer bis tiefer Hypothermie: Plasma-Katecholaminverhalten, Metabolismus und Kreislauffunktion. Anaesthesist 33, 311-315
23. Turner E., Hilfiker O., Braun U., Wienecke W., Rama: Metabolic and hemodynamic response to hyperventilation in patients with head injuries. Intens. Care Med. 10, 127-132

PROFOUND HYPOTHERMIA AND CIRCULATORY ARREST: STUDIES ON INTRAOPERATIVE METABOLIC CHANGES AND LATE POSTOPERATIVE INTELLECTUAL DEVELOPMENT AFTER CORRECTION OF CONGENITAL HEART DISEASE

J.A. RICHTER, R. KUNKEL

INTRODUCTION

Surgical and anesthesiological techniques utilizing deep hypothermia and total circulatory arrest (DHCA) have facilitated the primary repair of congenital cardiac anomalies in infants, allowing excellent surgical exposure and shortening the duration and complications of extracorporeal circulation (ECC). Dispite its worldwide clinical application, DHCA still remains an empiric technique. Many centers report improving results while others experience major problems as far as neurological complications are concerned. Correction and partial correction of congenital heart defects in DHCA, performed in the past ten years in the German Heart Center Munich, are demonstrated in table 1.

TABLE 1.

CORRECTION AND PARTIAL CORRECTION OF CONGENITAL HEART DEFECTS IN HYPOTHERMIC CIRCULATORY ARREST IN BABIES WHEIGHING UP TO 10.000 g

n = 941

APRIL 1974 – DECEMBER 1984

defect	< 1 Mo		1–3 Mo		4–6 Mo		7–12 Mo		> 12 Mo		TOTAL		
	n	†	n	†	n	†	n	†	n	†	n	†	† %
TGA	10	–	36	1	29	–	46	–	44	–	165	1	0.6
TGA + VSD	1	–	11	1	6	–	13	–	20	1	51	2	3.9
VSD	2	–	17	3	55	2	77	–	49	1	200	6	3.0
TOF	7	–	9	1	19	–	31	–	48	2	114	3	2.6
truncus	–	–	8	2	4	1	4	2	4	1	20	6	30
total AV–canal	1	–	5	1	10	1	28	2	20	–	64	4	6.3
TAPVC	22	3	17	1	7	–	5	–	1	–	52	4	7.7
valvular AS	27	7	12	1	5	–	3	–	3	–	50	8	16
complex defects	41	15	14	2	9	2	8	2	3	1	75	22	29.3
others	24	2	8	–	28	4	29	1	18	–	107	6	5.6
re–operation	4	–	5	3	9	4	11	–	14	–	43	7	16.2
total	139	27	142	16	181	14	253	7	222	6	941	69	7.33
mortality		19		11		7.7		2.7		2.7			
(+) = hospital. mortality (≤ 30 days)													

Recent studies from Treasure (1) show widespread neurological damage in animals after DHCA longer than 45 minutes. On the other hand, there is clinical evidence that a DHCA time of over 60 minutes at 16 - 18 °C in infants does not result in neurological or psychiatric disorder in most cases (8).

Steward reported the incidence of neurological dysfunction in a retrospective review of 218 patients less than two years of age undergoing DHCA at 18 - 20 °C at the University of Alabama, Birmingham (2). He found a 1.4 % incidence of coma and 2.3 % choreoathetosis. All these children were only core cooled and DHCA time exceeded 45 minutes. He concluded that surface cooling combined with core cooling might be safer by promoting a more even cooling of the organism. Most centers have abandoned surface cooling prior to core cooling in favor of core cooling with ECC alone. The question, which of the two cooling techniques is superior, is controversial.

The aim of our studies was to compare the two different techniques used to reach deep hypothermia at 18 - 20 °C core temperature, evaluating changes in systemic metabolism and trying to find a definitive answer to the question, which of the cooling procedures is optimal at least as far as whole body metabolism is concerned (3). A follow-up study of the neurological function and intellectual development 5 to 6 years after DHCA was performed, comparing the results of DHCA cases with those of a control group, which underwent cardiac operations using ECC techniques alone without DHCA (4).

PATIENTS AND METHODS

41 infants undergoing corrective surgery of congenital heart diseases were randomly selected in two groups. In the first group the body temperature was lowered entirely by perfusion cooling on ECC (ECC-C). There were 15 infants with a mean age of 9.4 months and a mean body weight of 6.11 kg in this group.

In the second group, representing 26 infants with a mean age of 7.23 months and a mean body weight of 5.5 kg, the combined method of surface and ECC cooling (SC-ECC-C) was applied. Profound hypothermia for circulatory arrest could be reached with both techniques.

TABLE 2.

DATA ON 41 INFANTS UNDERGOING DHCA WITH
1. cooling with ECC (ECC-C)
2. surface cooling + ECC cooling (SC+ECC-C)

	ECC-C (n=15)		SC+ECC-C (n=26)		
	x	+ SD	x	+ SD	P
Age (months)	9.5	7.3	7.2	5.2	0.13
Body weight (kg)	6.1	2.3	5.5	1.1	0.13
Surface cooling (min.)			56.0	12.0	
ECC cooling (min.)	11.6	7.9	8.5	3.8	0.05
CA time (min.)	36.2	19.8	46.7	15.8	0.02
ECC rewarming (min.)	55.8	31.6	49.7	27.7	0.23

The parameters measured in both groups are listed in Table 3.

TABLE 3.

PARAMETERS MEASURED IN BOTH GROUPS:

1. Arterial and venous blood gases
2. Arterial and mixed venous O_2-contents
3. Oxygen consumption during ECC
4. Arterial lactate level
5. Glucose concentrations
6. Electrolytes (Na^+, K^+, Ca^{++}, Cl^-)
7. Enzyme activities of CPK, HBDH, LDH, SGOT, SGPT

They were determined in either group as depicted in Table 4.

TABLE 4.

TIMETABLE FOR SAMPLES AND MEASUREMENTS:

1. After induction of anesthesia and during surface cooling (only blood gas)
2. from prime of the ECC-circuit prior to starting CPB
3. after starting CPB
4. prior to circulatory arrest
5. during CA in 10 min. intervals and at the end of CA
6. during the rewarming period in 10 min. intervals
7. at the end of the operation

Mean values and standard deviation were computed. Statistical analysis was further mady by Student's t-test utilising a 5 % level of significance.

In order to estimate the late psychological development of the infants, 21 children could be evaluated postoperatively five years after DHCA. 16 infants with similar defects, who had been operated upon during the same period by ECC alone without circulatory arrest, were randomly selected as a control group. The methods of evaluation are listed on Table 5.

TABLE 5.

ASSESSMENT OF INTELLIGENCE LEVEL

1. HAMBURG-WECHSLER-INTELLIGENCE-TEST FOR CHILDREN (HAWIK)
   Verbal + performance test - 5 subtests in each part
2. HEIDELBERG-LINGUISTIC-DEVELOPMENT-TEST (HSET)
   consisting of 10 subtests;
   Statistical analysis: "Statistic Package for Social Sciences" including Student's t-Test, Mann-Whitney-Test, Chi-Quadrat-Test
   $p < 0.05$

The psychologists who interviewed the parents und tested the children were not informed about the medical history, the type of operation and the ECC or DHCA techniques applied. The groups were comparable in family socioeconomy index, which was calculated using a weighted rating of educational and occupational levels of the head of the household. The influence of age, weight at operation, duration of DHCA and ECC as well as the influence of social index and other confounding variables on the subsequent intellectual development were explored using multiple regression analysis. For statistical analysis the "Statistical Package for Social Sciences" was applied.

RESULTS

I. Metabolic studies

There were no intraoperative complications related to cooling or rewarming in either group. The postoperative clinical course did not exhibit any difference between the two groups of infants.

Nasopharyngeal temperature averaged 21.3 and 22.8 °C in the ECC-C group and 20.5 and 22 °C in the SC-ECC-C group. Total cooling time was significantly longer in the SC-ECC-C group (64 min.). CA time was 36.2 $\pm$ 19.8 in the ECC-C and - significantly longer - 46.7 $\pm$ 15.8 minutes in the SC-ECC-C group.

The variations of metabolic parameters (pH, PCO_2, lactate, electrolytes, glucose, enzyme activity) induced by cooling, hypothermic circulatory arrest and bypass-rewarming were comparable in both groups. There were no statistically significant differences between the data obtained in the ECC-C and SC-ECC-C group.

In both groups a metabolic acidosis was present at normothermia, which was further aggravated during cooling. The extent of variation in base excess was not related to the technique of cooling used. The highest base deficit was measured 5 minutes after restarting bypass (-10.8 $\pm$ 6 ECC-C) v.s. (-13.5 $\pm$ 3.6 SC-ECC-C). Normalisation of base excess values occurred during the rewarming period.

The only statistically significant difference was found in $\dot{V}O_2$ during the course of rewarming on ECC.

Oxygen consumption was calculated from the data during total cardiopulmonary bypass. During cooling $\dot{V}O_2$ fell progressively and reached 2.77 $\pm$ 2.4 ml/min·kg in the ECC-C and 2.38 $\pm$ 1.7 ml/min·kg in the SC-ECC-C group immediately prior to CA. After restarting of the rewarming bypass $\dot{V}O_2$ increased to 5.17 $\pm$ 2.5 ml/min·kg (ECC-C) and to 6.08 $\pm$ 1.8 ml/min·kg (SC-ECC-C). This increase of oxygen consumption was followed by marked reduction in $\dot{V}O_2$ ten minutes after restarting bypass. With the rise of body temperature $\dot{V}O_2$ increased in both groups, reaching significantly higher levels in the ECC-C group: 5.02 $\pm$ 0.72 ml/min·kg (SC-ECC-C group: 3.29 $\pm$ 2.5 ml/min·kg).

II. Psychological observations

No statistically significant correlation was found between HAWIK/HSET IQ values and duration of ECC or circulatory arrest. The mean score of IQ in the DHCA group (113) was not significantly different from that of the ECC group (119) (Table 6).

TABLE 6.

HAMBURG-WECHSLER-INTELLIGENCE TEST FOR CHILDREN (HAWIK) and HEIDELBERG-LINGUISTIC-DEVELOPMENT TEST (HSET) mean total IQ scores

	DHCA-Group	ECC-Group	Norm in Population 50 % range
HAWIK			
1. IQ-Total	113	118	90-110
2. Performance	113	119	
3. Verbal	109	114	
HSET	47	51	47- 53

No deleterious effect on intellectual development could be demonstrated that might be attributed to DHCA or ECC.

DISCUSSION

The results of our studies confirm the findings of other investigators, that DHCA is a valuable method in connection of congenital anomalies in small infants (5, 6, 7). According to our results and the experiences of others the safe limit of CA-time at a NP and rectal temperature of 18 - 20 °C is about 50 minutes (8). In this series no operative death or postoperative neurologic complications attributable to failure of the methods were observed. The variations of metabolic parameters induced by cooling, DHCA and ECC rewarming were comparable in both groups of infants independant of the cooling technique applied. The higher level of O_2 consumption found in the ECC-C group during rewarming suggests that aerobic metabolism in peripheral tissues starts earlier than in the SC-ECC-C group. Initially less effective cooling of peripheral tissues by the ECC-C techniques, resulting in a higher temperature at the level of microcirculation, may explain this finding (20). However, the combined method of surface and perfusion cooling was seen to be more complex and time-consuming without any favourable effects on the outcome of the surgical procedure.

Published works on psychological development and intelligence quotient, subsequent to DHCA in infants for correction of congenital heart defects, suggest that no major psychometric impairment results (5, 6, 7, 9).

In our study IQ scores derived from the Wechsler Intelligence Scale for Children and the Heidelberg Linguistic Development Test were measured in 21 children five years following DHCA operations. The results of these patients were compared with those of a control group of 16 children with similar defects but operated upon using ECC techniques alone. The mean score of IQ in the DHCA group (113) was not significantly different from that of the ECC group (119).

No statistically significant influence of age, weight at operation, duration of ECC or circulatory arrest on total IQ could be demonstrated. Both techniques do not appear to cause neurologic dysfunction or impairment of intellectual development. The late mean IQ scores found were above the average of the norm in population.

Based on the results of our metabolic studies and psychometric testing it can be stated that ECC and DHCA techniques can safely be used in small infants undergoing intracardiac repair of congenital heart diseases. The beneficial protective effect of deep hypothermia on brain metabolism during circulatory arrest is evident since no adverse influence on subsequent intellectual development have been found, which could be attributed to the hypothermic techniques used.

REFERENCES

1. Treasure T, Naftel DC, C, Conger KA, Garcia JH, Kirklin JW, Blackstone EH: The effect of hypothermic circulatory arrest time on cerebral function, morphology, and biochemistry. J Thorac Cardiovasc Surg 86:761-770, 1983.
2. Samuelson PN: Pediatrics: Deep hypothermic circulatory arrest - what do we know? Society of Cardiovascular Anesthesiologists, 5th Annual Meeting. Abstract Boston, 1984.
3. Kunkel R, Hagl S, Richter JA, Habermeyer P, Sebening F: The effects of deep hypothermia and circulatory arrest on systemic metabolic state of infants undergoing correctiv open heart surgery: A comparison of two methods. Thorac Cardiovasc Surgeon 27:168-177, 1979.
4. Lange J: Intelligenz und Sprachentwicklung von 5-9jährigen Kindern nach Herzoperationen unter tiefer Hypothermie mit Kreislaufstillstand. Study for final examination in psychology, Ludwig-Maximilians-University Munich, 1983.
5. Cohen ME, Olszowka JS, Subramanian S: Electroencephalographic and neurological correlates of deep hypothermia and circulatory arrest in infants. The Annals of Thoracic Surgery 23, 3, 1977.
6. Brunberg JA, Doty DB, Reilly EL: Choreoathetosis in infants following cardiac surgery with deep hypothermia and circulatory arrest. J Pediatrics 84, 1:232-235, 1974.
7. Stevenson G, Stone F, Dillard DH, Morgan BC: Intellectual development of children subjected to prolonged circulatory arrest during hypothermic open heart surgery in infancy. Circulation, Suppl. II, 49:II54-59, 1974.
8. Wells FC, Coghill S, Caplan HL, Lincoln C, Kirklin JW: Duration of circulatory arrest does influence the psychological development of children after cardiac operation in early life. J Thorac Cardiovasc Surg 86:823-831, 1983.
9. Messmer BJ, Schellberger U, Gattiker R, Senning A: Psychomotor und intellectual development after deep hypothermia and circulatory arrest in early infancy. J Thorac Cardiovasc Surg 72:495-501, 1976.

FLOWS AND PRESSURES DURING CARDIOPULMONARY BYPASS

G.F. Karliczek

1. VISCOSITY OF BLOOD Flow of a fluid through a cylindrical pipe can be either laminar or turbulent . Friction with the wall of the pipe and the intermolecular forces, cause a typical velocity profile with the slowest speed adjacent to the wall. Ideally the flow profile has a parabolic shape in laminar flow, and a flat profile when the flow is turbulent (fig. 1).

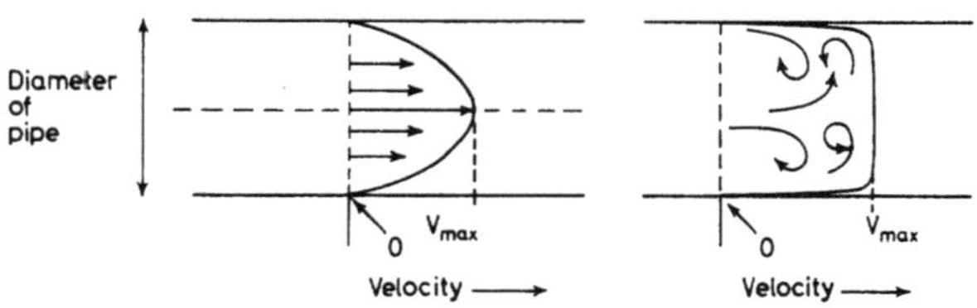

Fig.1: Flow profile in laminar or turbulent flow (from Hill [1])

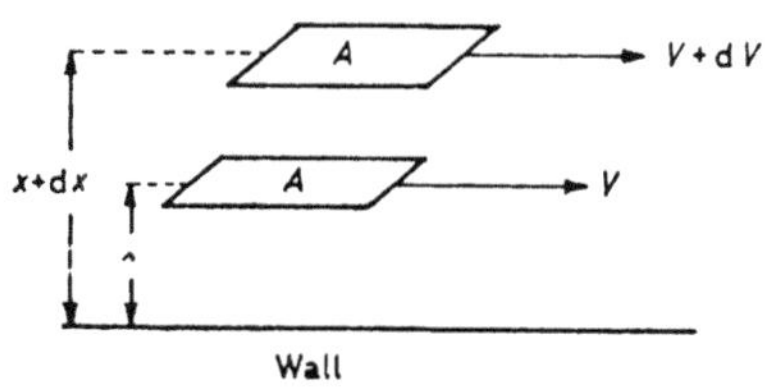

Fig.2: shear stress, shear force (from Hill [1])

$$F = \eta \cdot A \frac{dv}{dx}$$

Consider two parallel layers in the fluid with different velocities (fig.2).Due to internal friction in the fluid a tangential force,the SHEAR FORCE, will exist between them, this is "F" in our equation. The SHEAR STRESS is the force per area and has the dimension newtons per square meter. SHEAR RATE (or the velocity gradient) is the quotient tdv/dx, with the dimension s-1. The quantity n is termed the COEFFICIENT OF VISCOSITY of the fluid. The unit of viscosity is N s m-2 (Newton seconds/sq. meter) or POISE (P) in the c.g.s. system. The viscosity of water is 1 cP at 20 degrees. In a NEWTONIAN fluid shear stress is proportional to the shear rate (or velocity gradient) as shown in fig. 3. Blood does not behave as an Newtonian fluid. When blood flows slowly, aggregation and rouleaux formation occurs between the erythrocytes and this creates a fluid of high viscosity. As VELOCITY increases, the aggregates are broken up, and the blood becomes "thinner". Once all aggregates are dispersed a critical value is reached , above which viscosity remains unchanged as velocity increases. At low flow rates the viscosity of blood increases enormously, so that when blood stops flowing, a very high force is required to restart it. This is because erythrocytes are interconnected by negatively charged fibrinogen

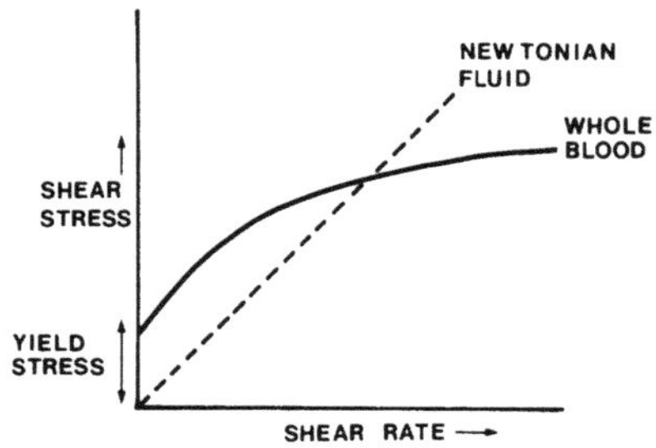

Fig.3: relation shear stress/ shearrate in NEWTONIAN fluids and in blood (redrawn from Gordon et al [2])

molecules at rest. The initial high force required to overcome these charges and set the system in motion is called the YIELD STRESS [2]. Other clinically important determinants affecting the viscosity of blood (fig.4) are the haematocrit, the concentration of fibrinogen and the temperature. Lowering the haematocrit from 37% to 17% will reduce the viscosity of the blood (at a shear rate of 125 s-1) by almost 50%. When the fibrinogen level is elevated this will increase the viscosity, particularly at lower shear rates.

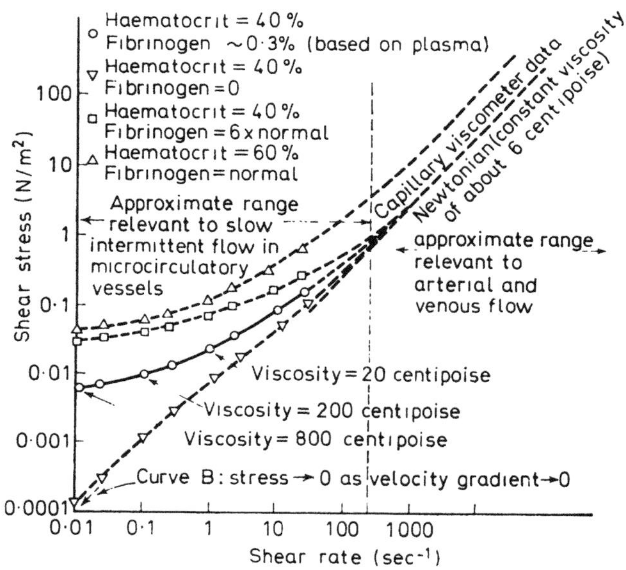

Fig.4: Shear stress against shear rate for bloods having various hct's and fibrinogen levels (from Replogl et al [3]).

When fibrinogen is elevated viscosity in the lower shear rates is markedly increased and nearly as high as the blood with a hct of 60%. Erythrocytes suspended in fibrinogen free slution behave like a newtonian fluid. In very small vessels (capillaries), viscosity at all rates of shear is lower than expected from shear rate. In these small vessels the red cells concentrate along the axis of the vessel, leaving a layer of plasma along the walls. Therefore the term "viscosity of blood" can not be applied in the microcirculation. The influence of the temperature on the viscosity of plasma and blood is shown in figure 5:

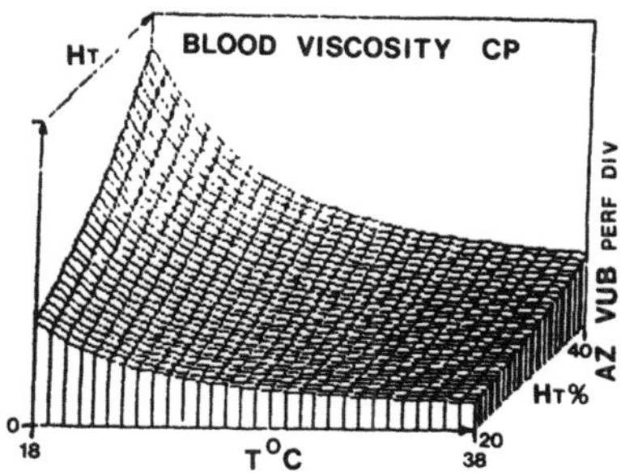

Fig. 5: Effect of haematocrit and temperature on blood viscosity (from Janssenwillem [4]).

As both temperature and haematocrit values undergo great changes during cardiopulmonary bypass, this will be reflected by changes of viscosity. These changed values of viscosity should not be neclected, when comparing values of peripheral vascular resistance. The formula to correct for changed viscosity is given in table 1:

$$SVR = \frac{\overline{AP} - \overline{RAP}}{CO} \times \frac{\eta_1}{\eta}$$

SVR = systemic vascular resistance
$\overline{AP}$ = mean arterial pressure
$\overline{RAP}$ = mean right atrial pressure
CO = cardiac output
η = normal blood viscosity at high flow at 37 °C (3·8 centipoise)
η_1 = viscosity of haemodiluted blood at measured temperature

Table 1: Systemic vascular resistance and viscosity (from Tobias and Fryer [5])

Naturally, patients with high haematocrit values, for example with congenital cyanotic heart disease, should not be cooled without hemodilution to avoid extremely high viscosity.

2. BLOOD PUMPS

During cardiopulmonary bypass (CPB), sufficient flow and pressure must be generated by a blood compatible pump. Numerous designs and constructions have been used, based on three different working principles: positive displacement pumps, kinetic pumps and closed volume pumps. The pump type in most frequent use is the roller pump (also known as Debakey's pump) (fig.6)

It is a closed volume pump. The rollers squeeze a tube, mostly of PVC or silicone rubber. The tube clamps with the bushings prevent the longitudinal movement of the tube, and the lateral escape movements are controlled by the guide rods.

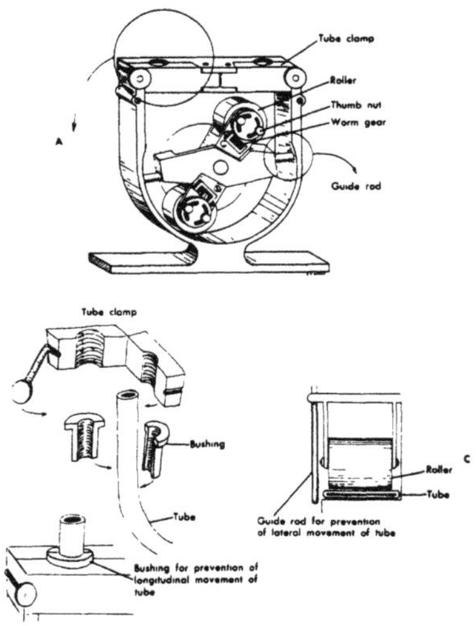

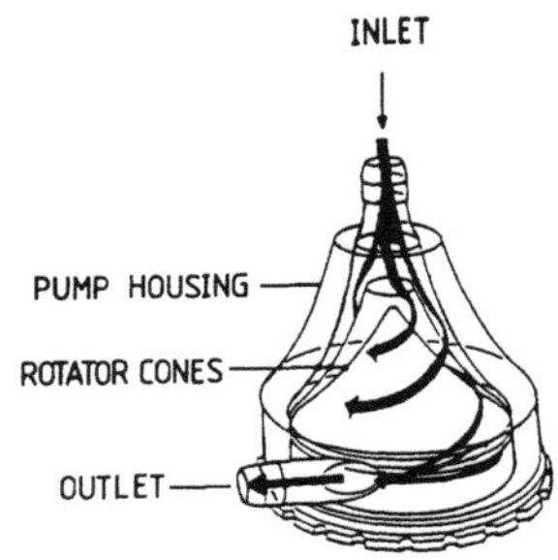

Fig. 6: Roller pump (from Nose [6])   Fig. 7: Biomedicus pump

The squeezing force of the rollers can be adjusted by a thumb nut to achieve an optimum of occlusivity. Total occlusion would mean that the formed element of the blood are squeezed between the walls of the tubing, and this is associated with severe hemolysis [7]. Alternatively too little occlusivity results in a high regurgitation rate with high shear stress. A shear stress higher than 150 N/m2 is reputed to to cause severe hemolysis. There are different methods to adjust occlusivity, which are not discussed here. It is important to remember, that the degree of occlusivity will change during the perfusion, due to changes of viscosity and plastic deformation of the tubing material. Roller pumps normally deliver a flow profile of almost steady flow and therefore the flow delivered by these pumps is nonpulsatile. Some roller pumps (such as the STOECKERT pump) can also deliver pulsatile flow.

KINETIC pumps are still very expensive and therefore rarely used for CPB. A typical example is the BIOMEDICUS pump. In action, blood passes through a vortex created by the spinning motion of smooth rotator cones. Occlusion of either inflow or outflow reduces or stops the flow. Large amounts of air entering the pump house will not be pumped, as it cannot develop enough centrifugal force to overcome the blood pressure in the outflow tube. This results in less hemolysis and platelet dysfunction than with a roller pump [8]. A further advantage is, that the pump is selfregulating in respect to preload. Besides the high costs there is the disadvantage that the output is dependant on afterload, thus electromagnetic or Doppler flowmeasurement is required. Kinetic pumps are therefore used for purposes outside routine CPB. Two synchronized BIOMEDICUS pumps have been used successfully as a temporary artificial heart [9]. It is also being used for veno - venous bypass in liver transplantation (without heparin)[10] and for left heart bypass without systemic anticoagulation for the repair of traumatic aortic rupture.

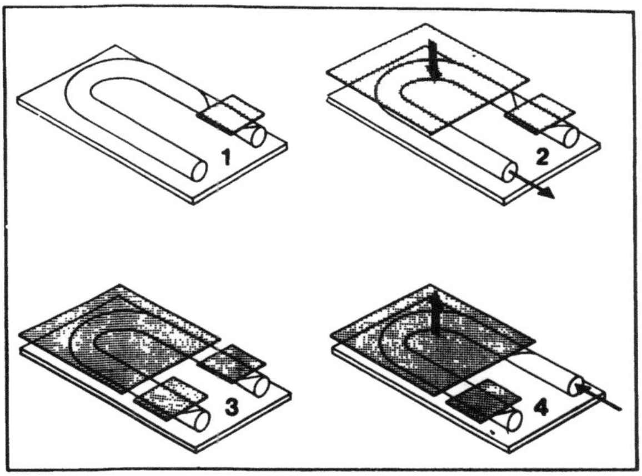

Fig. 8: Working principle of the Polystan pulsatile pump (from Hein [11])

An example of a POSITIVE DISPLACEMENT pump used for CPB is the POLYSTAN pulsatile pump. It lookes likes a roller pump - as it uses also only one piece of disposable tubing, but its pumping principle is completely different (fig. 8). It is designed only for pulsatile flow and has an an inflow and an outflow valve. However most commonly non pulsatile CPB is used, which is associated with numerous disorders of organ perfusion.

3. EFFECTS OF NON-PULSATILE BYPASS ON THE MICROCIRCULATION

Nonpulsatile flow leads to reduction of capillary blood flow and decreased flow of lymph and interstitial fluid [12]. It has been suggested by Burton [13] , that as the bloodpressure falls at the end of systole, blood flow in the microcirculation will continue until the critical closing pressure of the pre-capillary arterioles is reached, when capillary perfusion ceases. Burton suggests that the peak systolic pressure of pulsatile flow will ensure an effectively greater period of microcirculatory patency than equivalent levels of arterial mean pressures during non-pulsatile flow. Takeda [14] reported microcirculatoy shunting, widespread capillary collapse, capillary stasis and cell sludging with non-pulsatile flow; these abnormalities were prevented, when pulsatility was restored. Reduction of capillary perfusion due to capillary closure is associated with reduced cellular oxygen consumption, increase of lactic acidosis and reduced uptake of glucose. Besides these disturbances of the microcirculation CPB is associated with severe dysregulation of arterial bloodpressure which will have further impact on organ perfusion.

4. HYPOTENSION DURING CPB

Hypotension occurs at several times during CPB, and is frequent when bypass is initiated. A number of causes have been suggested for this initial hypotension: e.g. the fall in viscosity [15], dilution of circulating catecholamines [16], release of vasoactive amines, and a reduction of cardiac output as a result of too rapid drainage of the venous return before pump flow is adequate. It should be mentioned, however, that skilled perfusionists initiate CPB in most instances without a drop of pressure. Thereafter, rapid central circulatory cooling may lead to a centrally mediated depression of vasomotor tone with subsequent hypotension. This is regularly seen seen during deep hypothermia. Cardioplegia also leads to hypotension. This has two possible reasons: Firstly, when cardioplegic solution enters the systemic circulation it may also exert a "plegic" effect on the vasculature [17]. Secondly, the relaxed heart is extremely liable to distension. Luxation and distension of the heart may activate stretch receptors within the heart leading to reflex vasodilatation. Similar reflex-mediated hypotension may occur when the right heart becomes dilated as a result of poor venous drainage. Whether (fast) rewarming per se also leads to hypotension is questionable. But certainly there are events associated with the rewarming period that do cause aortic pressure to fall, for example: the release of the aortic

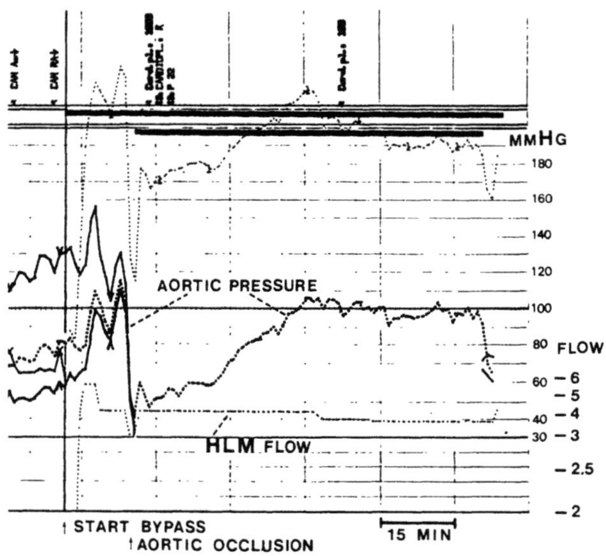

Fig. 9: Original anaesthesia protocol showing pressure and flow during CPB. Initially perfusion pressure is low and restores after some time on bypass.

cross clamp regularly leads to a fall in the aortic blood pressure. Also refilling with blood and removal of air often leads to abrupt distension of the myocardium, followed by reflex mediated hypotension [18]. Anaphylactoid reactions may be another, although infrequent, reason for hypotension during CPB.

5. HYPERTENSION

A definition for hypertension during CPB is non-existent. In most cardiac centra, however, a mean blood pressure higher than 100 mmHg during total bypass will be regarded as hypertension. Hypertension on CPB is most frequently seen in patients with a history of hypertension. But also normotensive individuals also tend to develop hypertension after some time (20 to 30 minutes) on bypass (fig. 9). This is due to a marked increase in the frequency of discharge of the carotid sinus baroreceptors [19,20] at the start of non - pulsatile perfusion. This in turn leads to neuro - endocrine responses and to reflex vasoconstriction in the peripheral circulation - either by direct neural reflexes or by stimulating the release of humoural vasoconstrictive substances e.g. the renin - angiotensin system [21,22]. Both the changes in the microcirculation and the bloodpressure dysregulation will lead to disturbances of the organ perfusion.

6. BRAIN PERFUSION DURING CPB

The literature on this subject has been reviewed by Simpson [23]. We know that cerebral perfusion is dependent on arteriolar tone. Autoregulation in normal man is maintained between mean arterial pressures (MAP) of 60 mmHg and 120 mmHg. Below and above these limits the circulation becomes "pressure passive" (Ingvar and Lassen [24]), i.e. varies with the MAP. Cerebral blood flow (CBF) was first studied by Halley and his colleagues [25]. They found, in dog experiments with nonpulsatile flow at constant

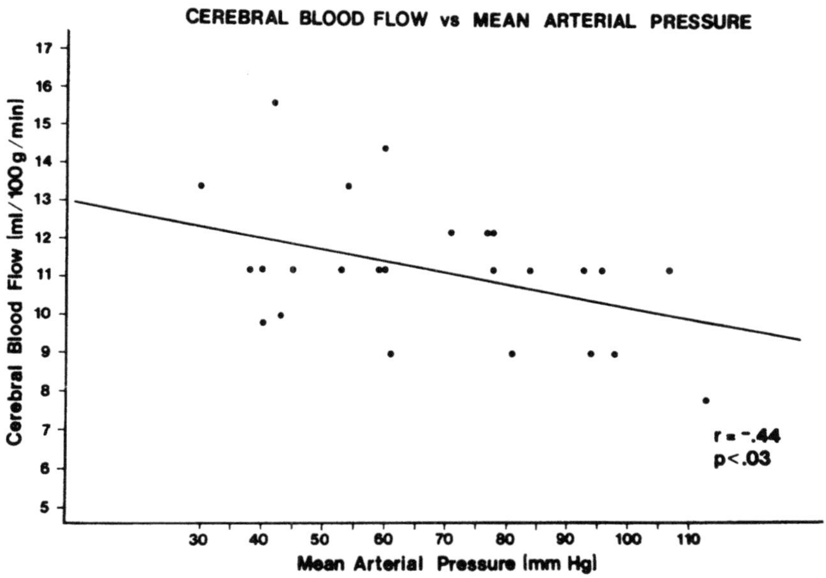

Fig. 10: Cerebral bloodflow vs. MAP during CPB in man (from Govier [28]).

paCO2, that cerebral bloodflow decreased when MAP became less than 55 mmHg and did not recover when MAP was raised again. However, an infusion of noradrenaline begun at that low pressure increased CBF dramatically. These results suggest loss of autoregulation at MAP 50 mmHg and developement of a pressure-dependent state with continuing low CBF. The assessment of CBF during CPB in man was first undertaken by Woolman and his colleagues [26]. They used cerebral A-V oxygen difference as a measure of CBF in patients undergoing nonpulsatile hypothermic (30 centigrades) bypass. They came to the conclusion that the $paCO_2$ was the most important factor influencing CBF under these conditions. Margaret Branthwaite [27] measured CBF with a jugular bulb thermo velocity probe. Her measurements were undertaken in the period of transition to CPB and during the first 15 minutes of nonpulsatile, normothermic bypass using haemodilution and with maintance of a constant $paCO_2$. The conclusion from her study was that the perfusion pressure was an important determinant of CBF and directly related to it. Recently, however, Govier, Mc Kay and Reves [28] have performed measurements of regional brain perfusion during hypothermic CPB under various pressure and flow conditions (fig. 10) and concluded that there was definiteley no correlation between MAP and CBF, it was deduced that autoregulation in moderately hypothermic patients under CPB is well preserved.

7. KIDNEY PERFUSION

During non pulsatile CPB, even at flow rates similar to normal cardiac output, renal bloodflow and glomerular filtration rate decrease [29,30]. The excretory function of the kidney, in particular, tubular sodium excretion, is impaired. There is also an increased release of renin, which is stimulated more by a decrease in arterial pulse pressure than by a decrease of mean arterial blood pressure. It is generally considered that the kidney stops working at a MAP of less than 50 mmHg. In individual cases it has often been observed that urinary production is maintained at MAP's below 60 mmHg. The critical closing pressure is 30 mmHg [31] in the kidney capillaries. MAP has no influence on postoperative renal failure according Abel et al. [32] and Hilbermann et al. [33]. Hence urin output is a poor parameter of adequate kidney preservation and lack of urine production does not mean renal damage.

8. The LIVER BLOODFLOW is normal with high flow perfusion [34]. With lower flows liver perfusion falls markedly; the a. hepatica flow is less reduced than the v. portae flow.

9. The SCELETAL MUSCLEs represents about 20% of the bodyweight. At rest (but not on CPB) the muscles receive about 8% of the cardiac output. During CPB this is probably much less. Laver [35] has demonstrated that the muscle mass cooles resp. re-warmes very slowly, and that one of the reasons for the temperature drop after CPB is that the muscles have not yet been thoroughly warmed. He therefore emphasized that temperature measurements should also be made in the muscle.

10. HOW MUCH BLOODFLOW DURING CPB? There is much confusion over how much flow should be given during CPB. The reason for this is that it would be an oversimplification to speak about "THE flow on CPB". Just as ventilator settings are adjusted during artificial ventilation according to various circumstances, the flowrate during CPB has to be adapted to various parameters such as metabolic rate, aortic pressure and surgical requirements.

10.1. METABOLISM

The influence of body temperature on metabolism is well known. Between 37-30 centigrades there is a 7% per degree reduction in O_2 consumption. But below 30 degrees, however, the reduction in VO_2 is non-linear and therefore less predictable. There is also the problem of defining the body temperature since there are large differences in the temperatures measured at various sites inside the body during cooling and re-warming. Muscle relaxation has an

important influence on oxygen consumption too. Insufficient relaxation during CPB can increase the oxygen demand to the limits of the oxygenating capacity of an oxygenator. Oxygen uptake during CPB depends also on the flowrate. Disturbances in the microcirculation during (non-pulsatile) CPB possibly explain why the the flowrate itself determines the oxygen uptake. Paneth and colleagues [36] have described the relationship between flow rate and oxygen consumption at low CPB flow rates .
When low flow rates are subsequently increased V02 increases. With greater flows this increase is less. A plateau is reached at a flow rate of 2.1 l/min/m2 and at greater flow rates V02 does not increase further.

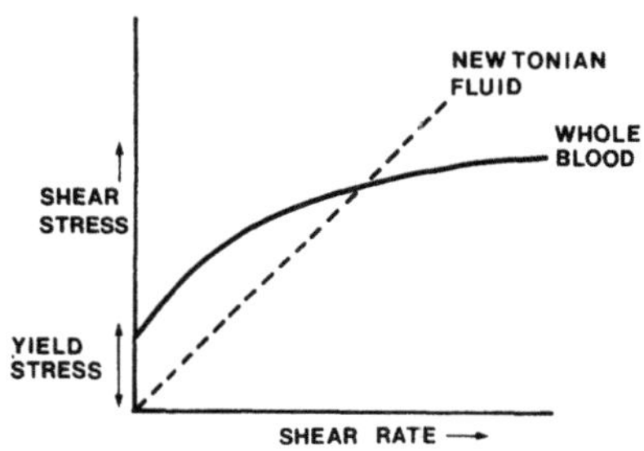

Fig. 11: Relation between 02 uptake and flow (Paneth [36])

The oxygen needs of tissues drained by the IVC are not met until the flow exceeds 1.2 l/min/m2, whilst the maximum oxygen consumption of the upper half of the body is reached with a 0.7 l/min/m2 flow rate [34]. A common parameter of the adequacy of the flowrate regarding the metabolime is the mixed venous oxygen tension (pv02). The mixed venous oxygen tension should

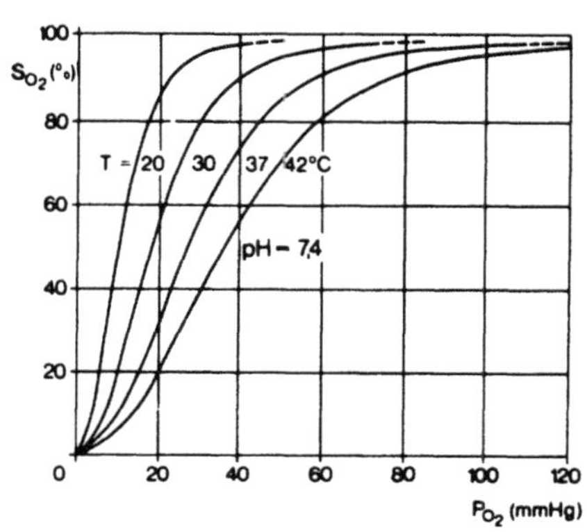

Fig. 12: Influence of hypothermia on the oxygen binding curve of haemoglobin (from Thews [38])

be greater than 40 mmHg (5.3 kpa); a pvO_2 value < 27 mmHg is reported to cause problems with cerebral oxygenation and < 15 - 18 mmHg not to be compatible with life [37]. In place of the mixed venous oxygen tension it is also possible to use the mixed venous saturation, which can be reliably measured with on-line oxymetry. When using the saturation, however one must consider the possible shifts of the hemoglobin dissociation curve, particularly that caused by hypothermia (fig. 12). In normothermia mixed venous saturation should be kept at or above 70 %, at 30 degrees at or above 80 %, and at 20 degrees saturation must be above 90 %. At low flowrates the oxygen saturations in two venae cavae can differ greatly and it is recommended that the flow be adjusted according to the lower svO_2 of the two. While low values of mixed venous oxygen tension (or saturation) clearly indicate that the flowrate is too low, normal or high values of oxygen tension (or saturation) can be misleading. In the presence of large AV shunts venous pO_2 and SO_2 may be high, whilst the capillary beds are poorely perfused.
Similarly a "normal" pH value is frequently advocated as an indicator for an adequate perfusion rate. A decreasing pH value certainly indicates that the flow is too low. The interpretation of the absolute pH value during hypothermic CPB is still problematic, as it is controversial which pH value should be used during hypothermia - the temperature-corrected value or the huncorrected value [39]. Metabolism is not the only determinant of bloodflow, numerous others factors require adjustment of the flow.

10.2. VARIOUS OTHER REASONS FOR ADJUSTING THE FLOWRATE

10.2.1. MYOCARDIAL PROTECTION

Conti [40] found that , when using a flow of 2.2 l/min/m2 and higher, it may be impossible to maintain the heart at a low temperature because of warming via coronary collateral flow.

10.2.2. NEED FOR DRY SURGICAL FIELD

A dry surgical field facilitates the surgery (better visability) and improves protection of the cardioplegic arrested heart. That is one of the reasons why cardiac arrest techniques are so populair in paediatric cardiac surgery.

10.2.3. LESS BLOOD DESTRUCTION

High flow results in much more blood being aspirated through the cardiotomy suction lines. When membrane oxygenators are used suction is the main source of blood trauma. Hence, reducing flow reduces suction and blood trauma [41].

11. HOW HIGH MUST THE BLOODPRESSURE BE DURING CPB?

The greatest fear of every clinician is that hypotension during CPB will result in neurological damage. Branthwayth's conclusion, that during bypass CBF is dependant on the mean aortic pressure, is supported by the clinical studies of STOCKARD [42]. He used a "Hypotension Index" [the time during which the MAP is below 50 mmHg in minutes x (50 - MAP) to quantify hypotension. He compared three groups of patients with different hypotension indices and found that neurological deficit was most frequently absent in the group with the smallest hypotension index. He therefore warned that hypotension (MAP < 60 mmHg) in normothermia is dangerous and concluded, that a hypotension index > 50 - 100 mmHg x min is hazardous for the brain. Possibly these results have led to the widespread opinion that MAP should be maintained during CPB. However this opinion is not accepted

		No deficit	Temporary deficit	Organic brain syndrome	Permanent deficit	Irreversible coma
	>600				①	①
Hypotension as tm^{50} / (50 mm	350–600			③	③	
Hg-MAP) δt in torr-minutes	100–350	•	⑥ ⑤ ④	⑤ ④	②	②
	0–100	•••••••••••••	••	•		

Table 2: Relation between perfusion index and neurogical disorders (from Stockard [42])

by everyone. Low flow, low pressure perfusion is advocated in several papers [35,43,44]. The arguments for low pressure, low flow perfusion are the reduced trauma to blood constituents, the dry surgical field, and better myocardial preservation via the reduction in cardioplegia washout. Despite low flow, low pressure perfusion the incidence of neurological damage and renal complications is reported in these papers not to be increased.

In addition Govier et al [28] have shown that pharmacologic treatment of MAP between 30 and 110 mmHg is unnnecessary, and that the recommmendation to maintain a perfusion pressure >50 mmHg cannot be defended on the premise that increased bloodpressure will increase cerebral blood flow. We ourselves allow the bloodpressure to fall to any value, in children and young adults provided the patient is hypothermic (< 25 degrees), the venous pressure is low, and the metabolic criteria (such as svO2 and pH) remain satisfactory. Nevertheless, we still have severe doubts whether prolonged severe hypotension is well tolerated in the elderly patients.

11.1. TREATMENT OF HYPOTENSION

There are two possible ways of increasing MAP: either by increasing flow or by increasing the resistance by giving a vasoconstrictor drug (e.g. cphenylephrine). Increasing the flow often fails, particularly in cases of reflex mediated hypotension (as described above), and may even worsen the situation. The venous canulae may be too small in relation to the increased flow resulting in further distension of the heart, and thus perpetuating reflex vasodilation. It makes sense, however, to increase the flow when this is indicated by decreasing venous saturation, decreasing urine flow or poor peripheral circulation.

11.2. TREATMENT OF HYPERTENSION

Vasodilator therapy is generally accepted in this situation. Among the recommended vasodilator drugs are sodium nitroprusside, regitine, and dehydrobenzperidol; others use halothane or isoflurane administered via the oxygenator. Reducing the flow is not appropriate, and the blood pressure will return to the elevated values a short while after the reduction of flow. However, when an acute reduction in the aortic pressure is reqired, reduction of flow is reasonable.

12. PULSATILE FLOW?

The technical problems involved in maintaining pulsatile flow during CPB have been solved [12]. There is some evidence that many of the severe disorders of the microcirculation and organ perfusion are attenuated or avoided if pulsatile flow is employed [12,37]. It has, however, still to be demonstrated whether pulsatile flow applied on a large scale in routine CPB will significantly reduce the morbidity associated with extra corporeal circulation.

References:

1 Hill DW: Physics applied to Anaesthesia, Butterworth publishers, London, 1972
2 Gordon RJ, Ravin M, Rawitscher RE, Daicoff GR: Changes in arterial pressure viscosity and resistance during cardio-pulmonary bypass, J Thorac Cardiovasc Surg 69,552,1975
3 Replogle RL, Meiselman HJ, Merill EW: Clinical implications of blood rheology studies, Circulation 36,148,1978
4 Janssenwillem, E: Registratie en verwerking van data tijdens extra corporale corculatie, NeSECC journaal,10,2,30,1985
5 Tobias MA, Fryer JM: Which priming fluids? In Longmore D: Towards Safer Cardiac Surgery, MTP press, Lancaster, England,1981
6 Nose Y (ed): Manual of artificial organs, Vol II: The Oxygenator, Mosby Company, St louis, 1973
7 Blackshear PL, Dorman FD, Steinmann JH: Some mechanical effects that influences hemolysis. Trans amer Soc Artif Int Org, Vol IX, 112,1965
8 de Jong: Cardiopulmonary Bypass, the effect on blood elements in dogs. Inaugural dissertation, Groningen, the Netherlands, 1985.
9 Dixon CM, Magovern GJ: Evaluation of the Bio Pump for long-term cardiac support without heparinization, J of Extracorporeal Technology, Vol 14, 2, 1982
10 McSteen F, Hackett J, Rhoades W, Merritt P: Heparinless Bypass for Liver Transplantation, Proc American Academy of Vascular Perfusion, vol 5, 28, 1984
11 Hein L, Green CG: Theoretical and practical considerations in designing a pulsatile pump. 16th internat. conference of the American Society of Extracorporeal Technology, San Diego, USA, 1978
12 Taylor K: Why pulsatile flow during cardiopulmonary bypass? In Longmore D (ed): Towards Safer Cardiac Surgery, MPT press, Lancaster, England, 1981
13 Burton AC: Relation of structure to function of the tissues of the wall of the blood vessels. Physiol Rev 34,618,1954
14 Takeda J: Experimental study of peripheral circulation during extracorporeal circulation with a special reference to a comparison of pulsatile flow with non pulsatile flow. Arch Jpn Chir, 29, 1407, 1960
15 Gordon RJ, Ravin M, Rawitscher RE, Daikoff GR: Changes in arterial pressure, viscosity, and resistance during cardio-pulmonary bypass J Thor Cardiovasc Surg 69,552,1975
16 Balasaraswathi K, Glisson SN, El Etr AA, Azad C: Effects of priming volume on serum catecholamines during cardio-pulmonary bypass Can Anaes Soc J 27, 135, 1980
17 Bretschneider HJ: Personal communication

18 Guyton AC: Textbook of Medical Physiology, 3rd ed, WB Saunders Company, Philadlphia and London, 1966
19 Angell-James JE, Burgh Daly M: Effects of graded pulsatile pressure on the reflex vasomotor responses elicited by changes of mean pressure in the perfused carotic sinus - aortic arch regions of the dog. J. Physiol. 214, 51, 1971
20 Harrison TS, Chawla RC, Seaton GF, Robinson BH: Carotid sinus origin of adrenergic responses comprising the effectiveness of artificial circulatory support. Surgery, 68, 20, 1970
21 Taylor KM, Morton JJ, Brown JJ, Bain WH, Caves PK: Hypertension and the renin-angiotensin system following open heart surgery. J. Thoracic Cardiovasc. Surg. 74, 840, 1977
22 Favre L, Valloton MB, Muller AF: Relationship between plasma concentrations of angiotensin I, angiotensin II, and plasma renin activity during cardiopulmonary bypass in man. Eur. J. Clin. Invest. 4, 135, 1976
23 Simpson JC: Cerebral perfusion during cardiac surgery using cardiac bypass. In Longmore D (ed): Towards Safer Cardiac Surgery, MPT press, Lancaster, England, 1981
24 Ingvar D, Lassen N: The human cerebral circulation. Acta Physiol. Scand. 62, 164, 1967
25 Halley M, Reemstra K, Creech O: Cerebral blood flow, metabolism and brain volume in extra-corporeal circulation. J. Thoracic. Surg. 36, 506, 1958
26 Woolman H et al: Cerebral blood flow in man during extra-corporeal circulation. J. Thoraacic. Surg. 52, 558, 1966
27 Branthwaite M: Cerebral blood flow and metabolism during open heart surgery. Thorax. 29, 633, 1974
28 Govier AV, McKay RD, Reves JG, Karp RB, Buttner E, ZOrn GL, Morawetz RB: Relationship of cerebral blood flow and perfusion pressure during cardiopulmonary bypass. Soc. of Cardiovascular Anaesthesiologists, Fifth annual meeting, San Diego, California, USA, 1983
29 Replogl RL, Gross RE: Renal function during ECC. J. Surg. Res. 1, 91, 1961
30 Utley JR, Wachtel C, Cain RB, Spaw EA, Collins JC, Stephens DB:Effects of hypothermia,hemodilution and pump oxygenation on organ water content, blood flow and oxygen delivery, and renal function. Ann. Thorac. Surg. 31, 121, 1981
31 Ream KE, Fogdall RP (eds): Acute cardiovascular management. JB Lippincott Company, Philadelphia, Toronto, 1982
32 Abel RM, Buckley MJ,Austen WG, Barnett GO, Beck CH, Fischer JE: Etiology, incidence and prognosis of renal failure following cardiac operations: Results of prospective analysis of 500 consecutive patients. J Thorac Cardiovasc Surg 71, 323, 1976
33 Hilbermann M, Myers BD, Carrie BJ, Derby G, Jamison RL, Stinson EB: Acute renal failure following cardiac surgery J Thorac Cardiovasc Surg 77, 888, 1979
34 Galetti PM, Breecher GA (eds):Bypass principles and techniques of extracorporeal circulation. Grune and Stratton, New York, 1962
35 Laver MB: personal communication

36 Paneth M, Sellers R, Gott VL, Weirich WI, Allen P, Read RC, Lillehei CW: Physiologic studies upon prolongend cardiopulmonary bypass with the pumpoxygenator with particular reference to 1) acid base balance 2) siphon caval drainage J Thorac Cardiovasc Surg 34,570,1957

37 Lake, Cl: Cardiovascular Anesthesia, Springer-Verlag, New York Berlin Heidelberg Tokyo, 1985

38 Thews, G: Atemgastransport und Saurebasen Status des Blutes in: Schmidt RF, Thews G (eds): Physiologie des Menschen, Springer, Berlin-Heidelberg-New York, 1977

39 Swan H: The importance of acid-base management for cardiac and cerebral preservation during open heart surgery. Surgery, Gynecology and Obstetrics, vol 185, 391, 1984

40 Conti VR, Bertanon EG, Blackstone EH, et al: Cold cardioplegia versus hypothermia for myocardial protection. J. Thorac. Cardiovasc. Surg. 76, 577, 1978

41 Boonstra PW, van Imhoff, GW, Eysman L, Kootstra GJ, Homan van der Heide JN, Karliczek GF, Wildevuur CRH: Reduced platelet activation and improved hemostasis after controlled cardiotomy suction during clinical membrane oxygenator perfusion. J. Thorac. Cardiovasc. Surg. 89, 900, 1985

42 Stockard J, Bickford R, Schauble J: Pressure dependent cerebral ischemia during cardiopulmonary bypass. Neurology 23, 251, 1973

43 Ellis RJ, Wisniewski A, Potts A, Calhoun C, Loucks P, Wells MR: reduction of flow rate and critical pressure at moderate hypothermia does not result in cerebral dysfunction. J. Thorac. Cardiovasc. Surg. 79, 173, 1980

44 Kolkka R, Hilbersman M: Neurologic dysfunction following cardiac operation with low-flow, low-pressure cardiopulmonary bypass. J. Thorac. Cardiovasc. Surg. 79, 432, 1980

PROMOTING CARDIAC METABOLISM BEFORE AND AFTER CARDIOPULMONARY BYPASS (CPB)

W.HAIDER, G.KRIEGER

1. INTRODUCTION

CPB is to be seen as a general stress state and therefore also a subject of a metabolic trauma to the organism. Moreover, during aortic cross clamping, a decrease of coronary perfusion and concomitant myocardial ischemia takes place.

With respect to stress an increase in catecholamine excretion, an insulin suppression and glucose intolerance - both leading to increased blood sugar level - and an increase in free fatty acid (FFA) serum level are noted.

With respect to myocardial ischemia a loss of diffusable adenine nucleotides is noted, thus limiting the AMP-availability and hence the ATP-recovery (1).

This situation can lead to an impaired myocardial energy production with a deteriorated sodium and potassium pump function and finally to "sick cell syndrome" with impaired cell membrane potential and cardiac performance.

2. METABOLISM IN STRESS

During stress a shifting of metabolism takes place from the most economic pathway of glycolysis towards lipolysis and also proteolysis. This seems to be primarily a useful "teleologic" measure of the organism, since in a 70 kg man the carbohydrate (CH)-stores amount only to approx. 350 g glycogen (=1.400 kcal), whereas the stores of fat amount to approx. 15 kg (=141.000 kcal) and the potential of protein to approx. 6 kg (=24.000 kcal).

With prolongation of stress, however, a number of disadvantages and limitations will occur:

The reduced CH-metabolism goes along with a persisting glucose utilization disorder with a lack of energy from CH; the increased fat metabolism leads to a rise in FFA serum levels, causing an increased myocardial O_2-consumption, increased incidence of arrhythmias and decreased myocardial contractility; and the increased protein breakdown might lead to nitrogen-catabolism with impaired cardiac function (2,3).

3. PROMOTING CARDIAC METABOLISM

A logic approach of influencing and promoting metabolism will be a back-shift of the deranged metabolism towards normal. Since energy metabolism (glycolysis, lipolysis) as well as protein metabolism is accessible by the hormone insulin, a simple way will be the administration of high doses of insulin together with adequate amounts of glucose and potassium.

The effects of insulin in CH-metabolism are enforcement of the intracellular glucose transport, activation of the phosphorylation of the glucose molecule and activation of glycogenetic (glycogen-synthetase) as well as glycolytic enzymes (phosphofructokinase, pyruvatkinase, glycerophosphatdehydrogenase, pyruvatdehydrogenase), thus stimulating glycogen formation as well as glucose utilization.

In lipid metabolism insulin develops an antilipolytic action and activates triglyceride-synthesis, thus decreasing the FFA-level.

In protein metabolism insulin develops its specific anabolic effect by increasing the cellular transport of amino acids and activating amino acid generation and protein synthesis.

In summarizing, insulin demonstrates exactly the opposite actions in shifting metabolic pathways than stress does (fig.1).

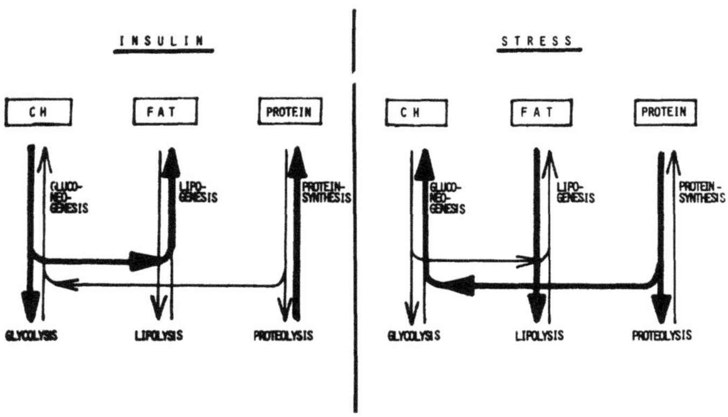

FIGURE 1. Opposite effects of insulin and a stress (shock) state on metabolic pathways.

4. INSULIN EFFECTS AFTER CPB

4.1. Shifting myocardial metabolism from lipolysis towards glycolysis

In patients following open heart operations, Moffitt et al. (4) showed significant lower serum levels of FFA and also of ketone bodies in an insulin treated group. In an own investigation (5) in patients undergoing open heart surgery, we again found in an insulin treated group significant lower serum levels of FFA as well as significant lower serum levels of cAMP, the central mediator in metabolism which to some extent reflects catecholamine activity.

4.2. Enforcement of the Na-K-pump mechanisms

In animal studies an insulin-induced increased Na-efflux and decreased K-efflux in skeletal muscle cells was demonstrated (6,7).

In an own investigation in patients undergoing open heart surgery (5), the patients after insulin administration showed decreased K-serum levels together with a significant decrease in urinary K-excretion, inspite of a doubled K-supply during the first 16 h, which obviously indicates an intracellular shifting of potassium (fig.2).

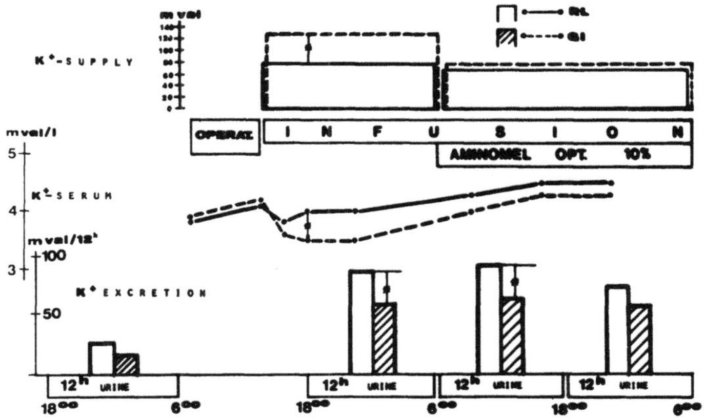

FIGURE 2. The effect of insulin administration in postoperative cardiac surgery patients on potassium serum level, urinary potassium excretion and potassium substitution (from Haider et al.; 5).

4.3. <u>Stabilization of the myocardial cell membrane potential</u>

Following the ideas of Sodi-Pallares et al.(8), who treated cardiac disorders with G-K-I as "polarizing solution", Zierler (9) showed in rat skeletal muscle cells an increase in resting membrane potential produced by insulin.

An indirect evidence of an increased cell membrane stability by insulin was shown by Hiatt et al.(10), who demonstrated survival with maintained sinus rhythm after an experimental left circumflex artery ligation in dogs receiving large doses of insulin, whereas all of the control animals died within 16 min in ventricular fibrillation (fig.3).

We found a decreased necessity of defibrillation after termination of CPB in an insulin treated group of cardiac surgery patients (11).

4.4. <u>Improvement of myocardial contractility and cardiac output</u>

In heart failure patients, Majid et al.(12) demonstrated an increase in cardiac output and dP/dt and a decrease in LVEDP by means of insulin. Rogers and coworkers (13) showed in insulin treated patients after myocardial infarction in contrast to a control group a shifting of left ventricular function in the field of a diagram constructed with cardiac index and pul-

Influence of insulin on circumflex artery ligation. (A) *Control (time recorded in seconds),* (B) *treated with massive doses of insulin (time recorded in minutes).*

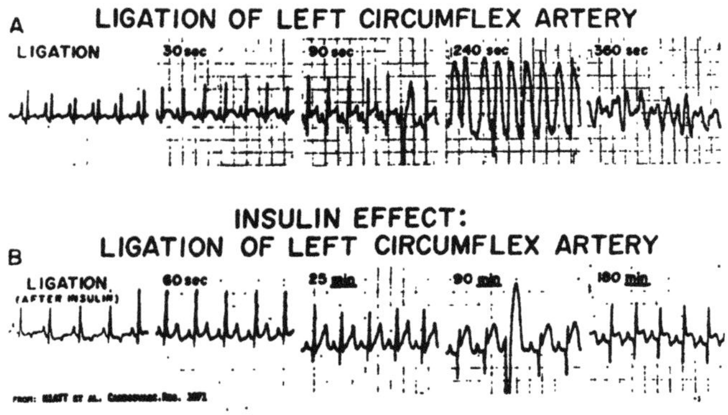

FIGURE 3. Insulin effect in dogs after experimental left coronary circumflex artery ligation: The animals in the non-treated group (A) all died in ventricular fibrillation within 6-16 min, whereas the animals in the insulin group (B) survived in stable sinus rhythm (from Hiatt et al.; 10).

monary artery end-diastolic pressure towards normal.

In patients following CPB, Moffitt et al.(4) found an increase in cardiac output by means of insulin. In an own study (14), cardiac output-measurements were undertaken in 20 patients immediately after CPB for coronary bypass grafting (fig.4).

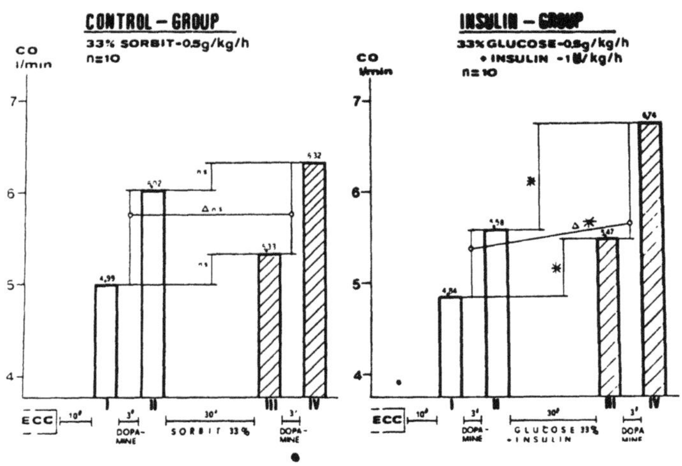

FIGURE 4. Insulin administration (1 U/kg/h) in cardiac surgery patients immediately after termination of extracorporeal circulation (ECC) causes a significant increase of the basal cardiac output (I vs.III) as well as a significant increase of the dopamine-induced cardiac output (II vs.IV) in contrast to non-significant changes in a control group with the same osmolar load (from Haider et al.; 14).

The cardiac output (Swan Ganz) was measured under basal conditions (I) and after a 3 min application of a dopamine challenge of 7 µg/kg/min (II). Afterwards during a 30 min period a control group received 33% sorbitol 0.5 g/kg/h, whereas the other group received insulin 1 U/kg/h together with the same osmolar load (33% glucose 0.5 g/kg/h). After this infusion period cardiac output was measured again under basal and dopamine-induced conditions (III, IV). In the control group the corresponding cardiac output values before and after the infusion period did not differ significantly. In the insulin group, however, the basal cardiac output as well as the dopamine-induced cardiac output after the insulin-glucose-infusion was significantly higher than that before the infusion.

All those data suggest that the metabolic intervention by insulin after CPB leads to a decrease of lipolysis and an increase of glucose utilization and to a consecutive enhancement of intracellular potassium shifting. This process obviously causes a stabilization of the cell membrane potential and on that basis leads to an improvement of myocardial contractility as well as to a better efficacy of therapeutic measures like catecholamine (dopamine) administration.

5. INSULIN EFFECT ON TERMINATION OF CPB

As described in a similar way also by Muller et al. (15), we found a facilitation in difficult coming off CPB. Also in patients who initially could not be weaned off CPB due to impaired ventricular function, it was finally possible to successfully terminate CPB after administration of insulin. In those patients, who seem to be untreatable massive doses of 20 U/kg insulin according to the data of Hiatt (10) were administered (fig.5).

6. INSULIN EFFECT BEFORE CPB (MYOCARDIAL PROTECTION)

6.1. Mechanism of action

Since myocardial protection from ischemic damage is normally achieved by decreasing the ischemic energy demand of the heart with cooling and cardioplegia, the preventive insulin administration represents an additional method of myocardial protection by increasing the ischemic energy provision to the heart. This will be due to a pre-ischemic manipulation of myocardial metabolism causing an enlargement of the myocardial energy charge.

The rationale of such a metabolic manipulation by preventive insulin administration prior to CPB is, that the myocardium's own ability to shift under conditions of reduced oxygen tension from oxydative lipolytic to anaerobic glycolytic energy sources represents an important survival mechanism (17). This is based on the fact that on the path of anaerobic glycolysis from glu-

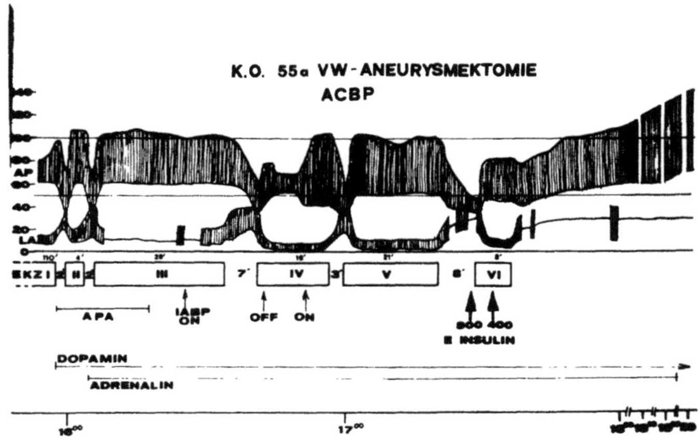

FIGURE 5. Course of arterial pressure (AP) and left atrial pressure (LA) during different unsuccessful trials to come off bypass (EKZ I-V) with pharmacological (catecholamines) and mechanical (IABP) support lasting 1 1/2 hours. After administration of massive doses of insulin (1.200 U)(at a blood sugar level of 550 mg% and a serum potassium level of 6.0) after 8 min the EKZ (VI) could be successfully terminated. Shown in a patient undergoind 3-fold CABG and anterior wall aneurysmectomy (from Haider et al.; 16)

cose to pyruvate 2 Mol of ATP are consumed (from glycogen to pyruvate only 1 Mol ATP), but 2 times 2 Mol ATP are produced, which amounts to a net gain of at least 2 Mol of ATP (from glycogen 3 Mol ATP) without oxygen.

An improvement of the myocardial survival conditions should occur if this metabolic switching - carried out by the heart in ischemia automatically - is anticipated, enlarging the myocardial glycogen depots prior to ischemia and ensuring the utilization of those depots during ischemia. Both actions are accomplished by insulin, since it enhances glycogenesis as well as facilitates glycolysis (see § 3).

Several trials have been made in the last 10 years by various investigators (17-23) using different methods in order to obtain better myocardial preservation by means of an augmented myocardial glycogen content. As summarized in fig.6, everyone of these approaches has achieved more or less of an increase in the myocardial content of glycogen and energy-rich phosphates as well as of an improvement in several inotropic parameters.

Since we had long been familiar with the administration of high doses of insulin in a therapeutic way, we tried to obtain enlarged myocardial glycogen stores by the administration of high doses of insulin in a preventive way.

AUSTEN ET AL. SURGERY, 1964	20 % GLUCOSE INTO AORTA	DOGS ECC	MYOC. GLUCOSE UPTAKE ↑	L.VENTRIC. FUNCTION ↑ (STARLING-CURVE)
SCHEUER ET AL. THE METABOLISM OF CONTRACTION, 1970	RESERPINE 24 H PRIOR TO PERFUSION	RATS ISOLATED PERFUSED HEART	MYOC. GLYCOGEN ↑ MYOC. ATP ↑	LVEDP ↓ DP/DT ↑
WEISSLER ET AL. CIRC.RES., 1973	INSULIN (100 MU/ML) INTO PERFUSATE	RATS ISOLATED PERFUSED HEART	AFTER 30 MIN ANOXIA: MYOC.CP ↑ MYOC.ATP ↑	L.VENTRIC. PRESSURE ↑ DP/DT ↑
HEWITT ET AL. SURGERY, 1974	FAT DIET 3 DAYS PRIOR TO ECC	DOGS ECC	AFTER 30 MIN ISCHEMIA: MYOC. GLYCOGEN ↑	CO ↑ DP/DT ↑
OPIE ET AL. CIRCULATION, 1975	GLUCOSE INSULIN (40-60 U/L) POTASSIUM 3 MIN AFTER COR.LIGATION	BABOONS LAD-LIGATION 10% MYOC. INFARCTION	MYOCARDIAL ATP 15% ↑ CP 15% ↑ GLYCOG: 25% ↑	INCIDENCE OF VENTRIC. FIBRILLATION ↓
LOLLEY ET AL. AM.ASS.THOR.SURG. 1981	GLUCOSE + FAT DIET OVERNIGHT	PATIENTS ACBP	MYOC. GLYCOGEN ↑	ARRHYTHMIAS ↓ VASOPRESSOR-NEED ↓
PASQUE ET AL. J.THOR.CARDIOVASC. SURG., 1982	RIBOSE - INFUSION PREOP.	RATS ISOLATED PERFUSED HEART	MYOC. ATP ↑	AORTIC PRESSURE ↑ CO ↑

FIGURE 6. Literature survey for different trials to obtain improved cardiac function by means of enlarged myocardial glycogen or ATP content.

6.2. Clinical and clinical-experimental data

In an own study (24) 20 patients undergoing mitral valve replacement received from the onset of anesthesia until the aortic cross clamping (average 80 min) insulin 1 U/kg/h, glucose 0.5 g/kg/h and potassium 0.25 mval/kg/h. After an average time of 26 min ischemia, a papillary muscle tip was excised and immediately plunged into liquid nitrogen determining ATP, ADP and creatine phosphate (CP).

The insulin administration was simply accomplished by using a 250 ml bottle of 33% glucose (82 g) with 160 U of insulin (Actrapid-NOVO), so that the relation g glucose : U insulin amounted to 1:2. The infusion was carried out with 40 gtt/min representing 0.5 g glucose/kg/h for a 70 kg man. The biochemical monitoring was carried out by the routine analysis of blood sugar and serum potassium.

The myocardial content of ATP remained significantly higher in the insulin group as well as the myocardial content of CP (fig.7). The calculated ATP/ADP-quotient was again significantly higher in the insulin group (5.19 ± 0.83 vs. 2.36 ± 0.52) as well as the energy charge potential (0.919 ± 0.009 vs. 0.851 ± 0.016).

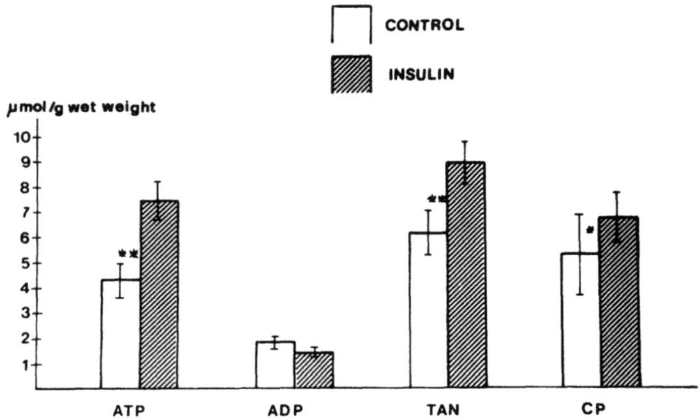

FIGURE 7. Postischemic content of ATP, ADP and CP in left ventricular myocardium of 2 times 10 patients undergoing mitral valve replacement with and without pretreatment of insulin. Significant higher (** $p < 0.01$, * $p < 0.05$) content of ATP and CP in the insulin group (from Haider et al.; 24).

The energy charge potential (ECP) which is a somewhat modified ATP/ADP-quotient, was described by Atkinson (25) as a cellular measure for either predominantly substrate synthesis (anabolism, high grade) or substrate consumption and utilization (catabolism, low grade) and was reported by Fürst et al. (26) as the "cellular expression for the capacity for biosynthetic reactions". It can be assumed therefore that the myocardial cells in the insulin group were in fact in a better energetic situation compared to those in the control group.

Because of the intracellular shifting of potassium by insulin, it was necessary to add until the morning of the 1st postoperative day a much greater amount of potassium in the insulin group (165 mval) than in the control group (102 mval) to keep the serum potassium level stable in both groups.

The increased lactate production with an augmented glycolytic flux is countered by infusion-cardioplegia during the entire aortic cross clamping time followed by good washout during the whole period of ischemia.

Because of the clinically most relevant question whether the higher myocardial ATP-content during ischemia is in fact of any hemodynamic benefit, we performed another study (27), investigating two comparable groups of 7 mongrel dogs each, undergoing experimental extracorporeal circulation (ECC) with 90 min aortic cross clamping time. Cardiac output (CO) by means of an aortic flow probe (Q_{aorta}) was recorded at different left atrial (LA) pressures of 5, 10, 15 and 20 mm Hg in order to construct left ventricular function curves. These data were registered prior to insulin treatment and onset of ECC (preischemic value), after termination of ECC (1st weaning off ECC) and after two 10 min periods of reperfusion (2nd and 3rd weaning off ECC). The 1st group served as control, whereas the 2nd group received high i.v. doses of insulin (total 25 U/kg) together with glucose and potassium within 60 min prior to the onset of ECC (fig.8).

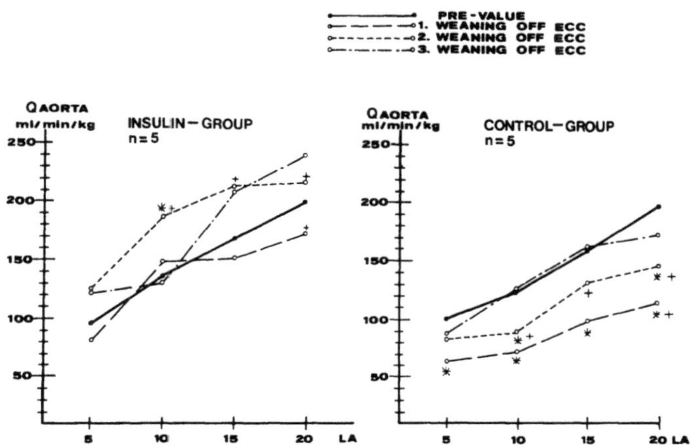

FIGURE 8. Left ventricular function diagram (CO vs. LA) and position of Starling curves (preischemic, 1st, 2nd, 3rd weaning off cardiopulmonary bypass) in two groups of 7 dogs each with and without pretreatment of insulin (from Haider et al., 27).

In the control group cardiac output after termination of the ECC and after the 1st reperfusion was significantly less than the preischemic value; only after the 2nd reperfusion (3rd weaning off ECC) it reached the preischemic range. In contrast cardiac output in the insulin group, however, was already within the preischemic range at the termination of the ECC (1st weaning off ECC). After the 1st and the 2nd reperfusion, cardiac output was partly even greater than the preischmic value.

This indicates that insulin pretreatment leads to an earlier postischemic restitution of a vigorous cardiac performance, suggesting better ischemic tolerance during aortic cross clamping. Again a much higher amount of potassium supply was necessary in the insulin group.

7. CONCLUSION OF INSULIN PRETREATMENT FOR MYOCARDIAL PRESERVATION

It is concluded that high insulin administration together with glucose and potassium before the onset of cardiopulmonary bypass leads to an augmented anaerobic utilizable energy provision for the myocardium (glycogen, ATP, CP) and a maintained cellular energy charge. Therefore a better myocardial cell function is maintained during ischemia causing a more rapid regeneration of the heart (Starling curves). This indicates preventive insulin administration a useful measure for an improved myocardial preservation from ischemic damage.

8. SUMMARY

The effect of therapeutically administered insulin together with adequate amounts of glucose and potassium in connection with a stress situation can be explained as follows: The metabolic effect of insulin causes an increase in glycogen storage and glucose utilization, a decrease in lipolysis and deleterious FFA-levels and an activation of protein- and enzyme-synthesis. Regarding the improved cellular energy, there are an optimal sodium pump and potassium shifting with stabilization of the cell membrane potential. This augmented membrane potential improves myocardial hemodynamics in a positive inotropic way.

The effect of preventively administered insulin can be defined as a production of an anaerobic available energy potential by means of an obvious enlargement of the myocardial glycogen depots and an increased and prolonged formation of energy-rich phosphates (ATP and CP) without oxygen. Since these effects imply preservation of the contractile performance following ischemia, improved myocardial protection is obtained.

REFERENCES

1. Pasque MK, Wechsler AS: Metabolic intervention to affect myocardial recovery following ischemia. Ann Surg 200:1, 1984.
2. Haider W: Vergleichende Betrachtung von Hämodynamik und Energiestoffwechsel im Schock. Anaesthesist 30:215, 1981.
3. Haider W, Semsroth M: Der Stoffwechsel im Schock und seine therapeutische Beeinflußbarkeit. Naturwissenschaften 68:583, 1981.
4. Moffitt EA, Molnar GD, Pluth JR, White RD, McGoon DC: Effects on metabolism and cardiac output of glucose-potassium solution with and without insulin. Ann Thorac Surg 15:1, 1973.
5. Haider W, Benzer H, Coraim F, Khosropour R, Mohl W, Müller M: Postoperative Therapie durch Akute Parenterale Alimentation (APA) mittels hoher Dosen von Insulin und Glukose nach Operationen mit der Herz-Lungen-Maschine. Anaesthesist 30:53, 1981.
6. Moore RD: Effect of insulin upon the sodium pump in frog skeletal muscle. J Physiol 232:23, 1973.
7. Zierler KL: Possible mechanisms of insulin action on membrane potential and ion fluxes. Am J Med 40:735, 1966.
8. Sodi-Pallares D, Testelli MR, Fishleder BJ, Bisteni A, Medrano GA, Friedlang Ch, de Micheli A: Effects of an intravenous infusion of a potassium-glucose-insulin solution on the electrocardiographic signs of myocardial infarction. Amer J Cardiol 9:166, 1962.
9. Zierler, KL: Increase in resting membrane potential of skeletal muscle produced by insulin. Science 126:1067, 1957.

10. Hiatt N, Sheinkopf JA, Warner NE: Prolongation of survival after circumflex artery ligation by treatment with massive doses of insulin. Cardiovasc Res 5:48, 1971.
11. Haider W: Prevention of stress reactions by influencing energy metabolism using the extracorporeal circulation as a model. Wien Klin Wochensch 87(Suppl):1, 1975.
12. Majid PA, Meeran MKM, Sharma B, Taylor SH: Insulin and glucose in the treatment of heart failure. Lancet IV:937, 1972.
13. Mantle JA, Rogers WJ, Smith LR, McDaniel HG, Papapietro SE, Russell RO, Rackley CE: Clinical effects of glucose-insulin-potassium on left ventricular function in acute myocardial infarction: Results from a randomized clinical trial. Am Heart J 102:313, 1981.
14. Haider W, Coraim F, Duma I, Eckersberger F, Kassal H, Semsroth M: Effect of insulin on cardiac output after open heart surgery. Anaesthesist 30:350, 1981.
15. Muller JE, Mochizuki S, Koster JK, Collins JJ Jr, Cohn LH, Neely JR: Insulin therapy for depressed myocardial contractility after prolonged ischemia. Am J Cardiol 41:1215, 1978.
16. Haider W, Benzer H, Coraim F, Wolner E: Massive insulin application as treatment in cardiogenic shock. Intensivmedizin 17:159, 1980.
17. Weissler AM, Altschuld RA, Gibb LE, Pollack ME, Kruger FA: Effect of insulin on the performance and metabolism of an anoxic isolated perfused rat heart. Circ Res 32:108, 1973.
18. Austen WG, Greenberg JJ, Piccinini JC: Myocardial function and contractile force affected by glucose loading of the heart during anoxia. Surgery 67:839, 1965.
19. Scheuer J: Some metabolic approaches to improving myocardial performance during cardiac hypoxia. In: Roy PE, Rona G(eds) The metabolic contractions. University Park Press, Baltimore, pp 195-207, 1975.
20. Hewitt RL, Lolley DM, Adrouny GA, Drapanas TH: Protective effect of glycogen and glucose on the anoxic arrested heart. Surgery 75:1, 1974.
21. Opie LH, Brynell K, Owen P: Effects of glucose, insulin and potassium infusion on tissue metabolic changes within first hour of myocardial infarction in the baboon. Circulation 52:49, 1975.
22. Lolley DM, Ray JF III, Myers WO, Sautter RD, Tewksbury DA: Importance of preoperative myocardial glycogen levels in human cardiac preservation. J Thor Cardiovasc Surg 78: 678, 1979.
23. Pasque MK, Spray TL, Pellom GL, Van Trigt P, Peyton RB, Currie WD, Wechsler AS: Ribose enhanced myocardial recovery following ischemia in the isolated working rat heart. J Thorac Cardiovasc Surg 83:390, 1982.
24. Haider W, Benzer H, Schütz W, Wolner E: Improvement of cardiac preservation by preoperative high insulin supply. J Thorac Cardiovasc Surg 88, 294, 1984.
25. Atkinson DE: The energy charge of the adenylate pool as a regulator parameter. Interaction with feedback modifiers. Biochemistry 7:4030, 1968.

26. Fürst P, Bergström J, Vinnars E, Schildt B, Holmström B: Intracellular amino acids and energy metabolism in catabolic patients with regard to muscle tissue. In: Johnston IDA(ed) Advances in parenteral nutrition. MTP-Press, Lancaster, pp 85, 1978.
27. Haider W, Eckersberger F, Wolner E: Preventive insulin administration for myocardial protection in cardiac surgery. Anesthesiology 60:422, 1984.

CORNARY CIRCULATION AND MYOCARDIAL METABOLISM DURING ANAESTHESIA*

H. SONNTAG, R. LARSEN, H. STEPHAN
Department of Anaesthesiologie - University of Göttingen, W.-Germany

To provide a basis for understanding and interpretation of the effects of anaesthesia first a brief review is presented of normal myocardial blood flow and metabolism and the alterations brought about by myocardial ischemia. In addition data will be presented from clinical investigations about the actions of anaesthetics on myocardial metabolism and coronary blood flow in patients with and without coronary artery disease.

Usually, the dynamics of the cardiac muscle are divided into three phases: those of energy supply, energy storage and utilization of energy.

In this text emphasis will be on the various substrates which provide an energy supply for the heart resulting in the formation of high-energy phosphate, adenosin triphosphate (ATP) and creatine phosphate (CP).
Under physiological conditions cardiac energy demands are exclusively met by aerobic metabolism, mainly of free fatty acids, glucose, and lactate, while breakdown of aminoacids and ketone bodies is of little importance. The energy supplying substrates are interchangeable. In normal oxydative metabolism, the most efficient process of cardiac energy production is, regardless of whether free fatty acids or glucose are oxydated, the Krebs or tricarbocylic acid cycle.

In the postabsorptive state free fatty acids supply up to 70% of the energy requirements of the heart by undergoing oxydative breakdown via the Krebs cycle. The uptake of free fatty acids by the cardiac cell is directly proportional to their concentration in the arterial blood, myocardial extraction being inhibited when the arterial concentration falls below 350 µmol/l.

At rest oxydation of carbohydrates accounts for up to 35% of the energy requirements of the heart, myocardial uptake of glucose depending on arterial concentration and the level of insulin. The uptake of glucose can be increased, when the arterial concentration of free fatty acids is low, also by increased metabolic demands and by hypoxia.
The following relations of myocardial metabolism of glucose and free fatty acids are of clinical importance:
- free fatty acids and their oxydative breakdown inhibit glycogenolysis and the uptake of glucose by the cardiac cell
- they also inhibit anaerobic glycolysis and oxidation of pyruvate
- while glucose uptake can be improved by the administration of insulin, myocardial glucose metabolism remains inhibited by free fatty acids.

Lactate is also consumed by the myocardium, the uptake by the cardiac

cell depending on sufficiently high arterial concentrations, since the cardiac cell membrane is not freely permeable to lactate.
The importance of oxidative phosphorylation for the metabolic integrity of the myocardium or the exquisite dependence of myocardial viability on the availability of oxygen are most obvious with hypoxia or ischaemia, which might occur during anaesthesia and surgery.

Hypoxia is a state of reduced oxygen supply to the myocardium despite adequate or increased coronary blood flow, while myocardial ischaemia is a restiction of coronary perfusion leading to myocardial oxygen deprivation and inadequate removal of metabolites.

The effects of a lack of oxygen on myocardial metabolism can be summarized as follows: During hypoxia the uptake and oxidation of free fatty acids are inhibited, while glucose uptake and glycogenolysis are stimulated initially. Anaerobic glycolysis of glucose by the Embden Meyerhof pathway becomes the only source of energy, leading to a decline on the rate of ATP synthesis and high energy phosphate and tissue glycogen stores. However, anaerobic metabolism can only supply as much as 10-15% of the high energy ATP that is formed in the well oxygenated heart. This amount is not sufficient to maintain normal contraction of the myocardium. In addition, in the ischaemic working myocardium the concentration of lactic acid and intracellular hydrogen ions rises rapidly, while in contrast, in the hypoxic well perfused heart washout of the acid products of glycolysis is maintained, thus retarding the rate of development of intracellular acidosis.

Myocardial metabolism is closely related to myocardial contraction and thus mainly depends on heart rate, peak wall stress, stroke work and calcium release and retrieval.
Also cardiac metabolism demonstrates a close coupling between coronary blood flow and myocardial energy requirements, i.e. coronary blood flow adjusts automatically to myocardial energy requirements. Under conditions of increased myocardial energy demand coronary blood flow rises in proportion to myocardial metabolism due to an unknown regulatory mechanism of the coronary circulation.
It is well known and has been recognized in current clinical anaesthesia, that myocardial oxygen demand and consequently coronary blood flow largery depend on haemodynamic determinants, which are summarized in figure 1.

Fig. 1

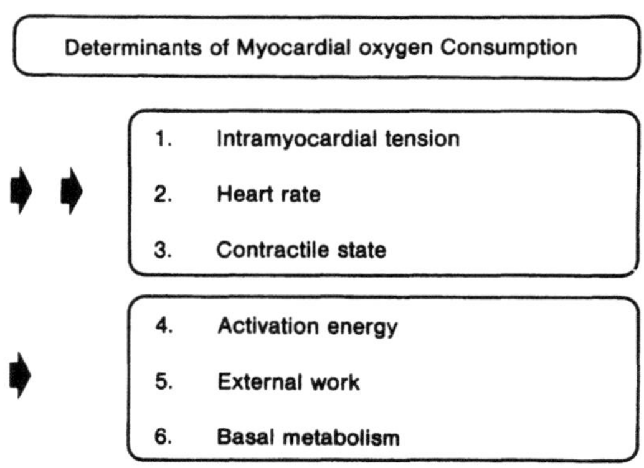

Of these, the first three parameters are the major determinants of myocardial oxygen consumption and metabolism, while the remaining only account for a minor portion.

Coronary blood flow is determined by the driving pressure and the coronary resistance, according to the equation given in the following formula: Coronary blood flow equals arteriovenous pressure gradient divided by resistance $(MBF = \frac{\Delta P}{R})$.
Traditionally, coronary perfusion pressure is calculated as mean diastolic aortic pressure minus left ventricular enddiastolic pressure or pulmonary wedge pressure. As will be shown later this assumption is not entirely accurate, particularly in patients with coronary artery stenosis.

According to KLOCKE coronary resistance can be divided into three functional components: basal viscous resistance, autoregulatory resistance and compressive resistance.
- basal viscous resistance is the impedance to flow during maximal vasodilation of the entire coronary vascular bed
- while autoregulatory resistance decribes the impedance to blood flow from the arteriolar muscle tone
- compressive resistance is the impedance to flow from intramyocardial tissue pressure which compresses the coronary vessels during the cardiac cycle and leads to a transmural gradient, which is greater in the subendocardial region than in the subepicardium.

Therefore, coronary resistance can be expressed in the following way:

$$CVR = \frac{P}{R_1+R_2+R_3}$$

this equation can be applied to both systole and diastole, with the contribution of each component to total coronary resistance changing throughout the cardiac cycle.

The compressive resistance is three to four times greater in systole than in diastole, while autoregulatory resistance is less in the subendocardial region than in the subepicardium during diastole, thus compensating the diminished flow to the subendocardium during systole.

During systole the intramural coronary vessels are compressed by the high intramyocardial pressures and coronary inflow is diminished, while coronary venous outflow is increased. In diastole intramural vessels are more distended by aortic mean diastolic pressure: coronary inflow increases, while venous outflow is decreased. As coronary perfusion pressure is decreased, for example by anaesthetics or as myocardial energy requirements are increased, for example by an increase in heart rate, blood pressure or intramyocardial wall tension, coronary blood flow is adjusted by autoregulatory vasodilation.

In the normal heart coronary blood flow can increase 5 to 6 fold without a change in coronary perfusion pressure, a phenomenon which is called coronary reserve. This is an inherent regulatory mechanism of the coronary circulation which decreases coronary vascular resistance to adjust coronary blood flow to the demands for oxygen. Coronary reserve has been defined by BRETSCHNEIDER as the ratio between coronary vascular resistance at rest and that during maximal vasodilation. In patients

with coronary artery disease, automatic adjustment of myocardial blood flow to myocardial energy requirements is diminished due to atheroma within the coronary vessels, increasing the vascular component of coronary resistance.
These relations are shown in figure 2 from LOWENSTEIN and co-workers.

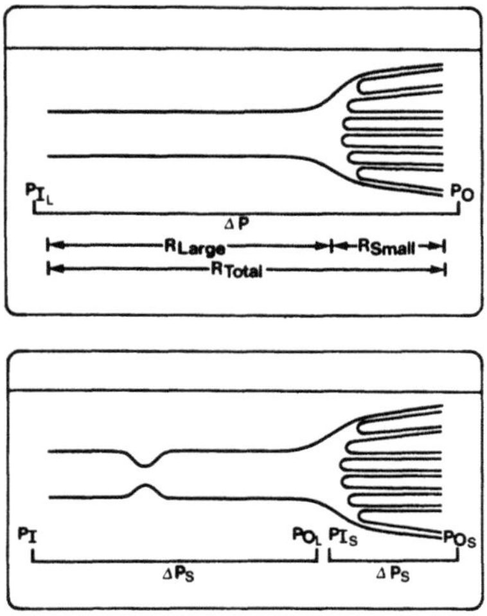

Fig. 2

The figure above demonstrates a normal vascular unit, the figure below a unit supplied by a narrowed coronary artery. Total resistance (R_{Total}) is the sum of the resistance of the large extramural and small intramyocardial vessels. In the normal unit coronary blood flow is determined by autoregulation. Perfusion pressure is the difference between the inflow pressure (P_I) and the outflow pressure (P_O). In the presence of a severe coronary stenosis, there will be a pressure gradient across the narrowing (P_{ILOL}). For this reason the small vessel bed is not exposed to P_{IL}, thus P_{OL} represents the inflow pressure to the small vessel bed (P_{IS}). Since the small vessel bed is assumed to be dilated completely with ischaemic heart disease, the pressure flow characteristics of the stenotic area determine the blood flow to the small vessel bed. In addition to the effects of stenosis the compressive component of coronary resistance might also be increased due to an increase in diastolic intramyocardial pressure further diminishing perfusion of the subendocardial region.

Heart rate may also influence coronary resistance in patients with coronary artery disease. In these patients the rate of shortening of the contractile elements cannot be increased, also, the rate of muscular relaxation is delayed, so that systolic time is increased at the expense of diastole. Thus the decreased time of myocardial perfusion impairs myocardial oxygen supply.

The severity of coronary artery disease is characterized more by a reduction of coronary reserve than by an impairment of coronary perfusion at rest, as is shown in figures 3 and 4.

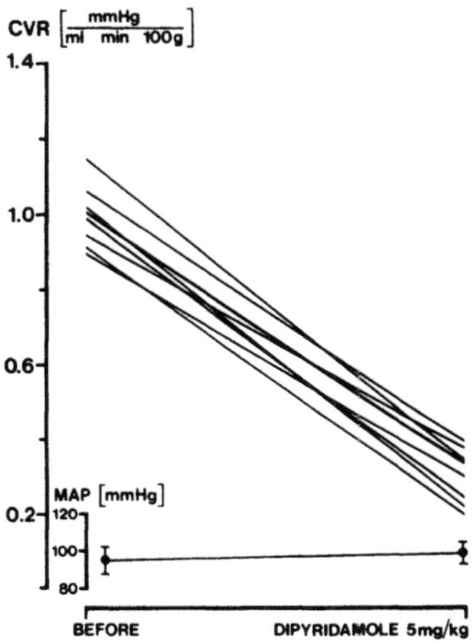

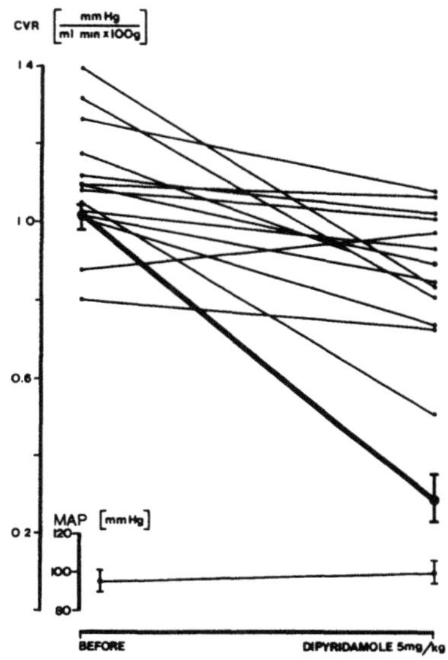

Fig. 3

Fig. 4

Figure 3 demonstrates coronary reserve in seven healthy patients. Coronary reserve was determined at rest and during coronary vasodilation induced with dipyridamole. Figure 4 shows the effects of vasodilatation in 12 patients with coronary artery disease. The intensified line represents the mean values of the healthy patients. Myocardial blood flow and coronary vascular resistance were normal at rest in both groups but the response to dipyridamole was diminished in patients with coronary artery disease, indicating that with the patients at rest, poststenotic arteriolar dilatation largerly compensated for the increased resistance in the extramural arteries. These relations indicate, that during anaesthesia and surgery rapid deterioration of cardiac function may occur when myocardial oxygen demand is increased but cannot be met due to impaired coronary reserve.

After a brief summary of the coronary and myocardial effects of anaesthetics in healthy subjects, the actions of inhalation anaesthetics on coronary circulation and myocardial metabolism in patients with coronary artery stenosis will be reviewed in some detail.
Since cardiac metabolism demonstrates a close coupling between coronary blood flow and myocardial energy requirements, one might expect that most anaesthetics affect myocardial metabolism and coronary blood flow due to their influence on the major determinants of myocardial energy demand. In fact, previous investigations by our group on the influence of various intravenous anaesthetics on myocardial metabolism in healthy volunteers (fig. 5) did not reveal any specific effect on myocardial

metabolism. With all anaesthetics free fatty acids remained the primary substrate for cardiac energy demand. All changes in coronary blood flow, myocardial oxygen consumption and metabolism were secondary to drug-induced changes in the haemodynamic determinants of myocardial oxygen demand (fig. 6). Similar results have been obtained with inhalation anaesthetics.

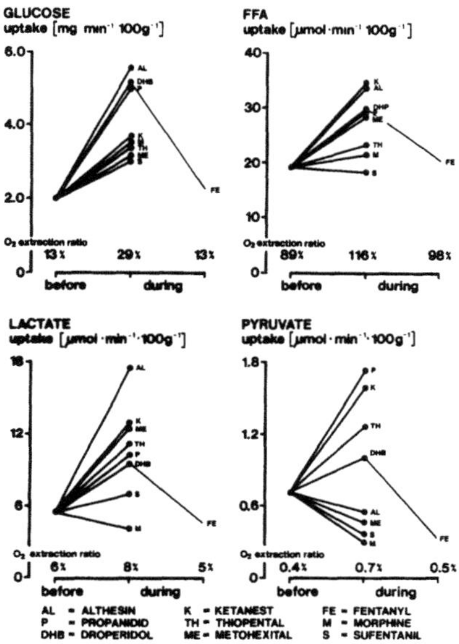

Fig. 5

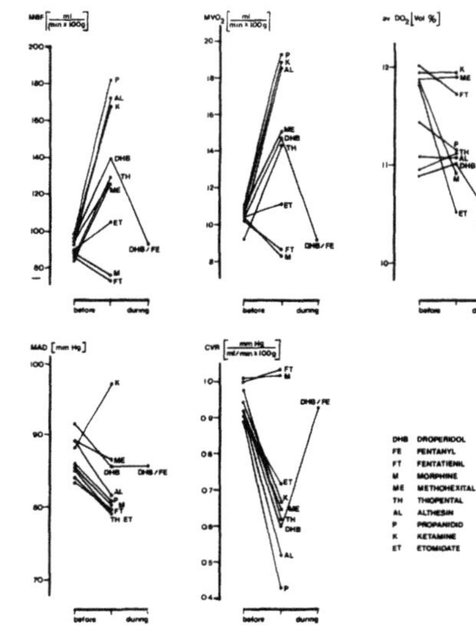

Fig. 6

Direct effects of anaesthetics on myocardial metabolism appear not to play a major role, rather, the effects of inhalational anaesthetics on overall myocardial substrate uptake in the non-ischaemic heart are predominantly related to effects of anaesthetics on cardiac function and hence on myocardial energy demand.

There are few clinical investigations concerning the effects intravenous and inhalational anaesthetics on myocardial metabolism in human subjects with coronary artery disease, and all animal studies have been hampered by the lack of a model of chronic atheromatosis. Also, it has been emphasized, that in view of the complexities of coronary circulatory control, experimental data are difficult of extrapolate to other experimental conditions and much less to human subjects. In addition, analysis of any specific effect of anaesthetics might be aggrevated by alterations in myocardial metabolism due to intraoperative episodes of myocardial ischaemia, which are unrelated to the anaesthetic technique.
The following figures show data from investigations by our group on the effects of various anaesthetic techniques on the coronary circulation and myocardial metabolism in patients undergoing coronary artery surgery. Measurements were performed with the patients awake (I), 20 min after

induction of anaesthesie (II) and during sternotomy (III).
Figure 7 demonstrates that the three anaesthetics did not produce major changes in heart rate. The mean arterial pressure was reduced to the same degreee in all groups after induction, while during sternotomy preinduction levels were reached again (fig. 8). Cardiac output was also reduced, the effect beeing less pronounced with isoflurane (fig. 9). Similar changes were observed in stroke volume index (fig. 10).

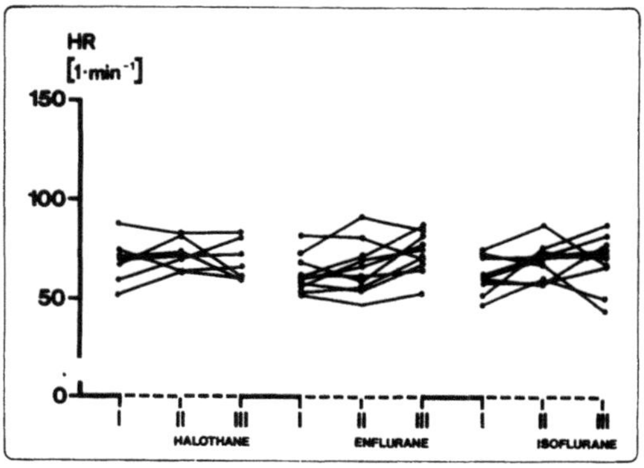

Fig. 7

Fig. 8

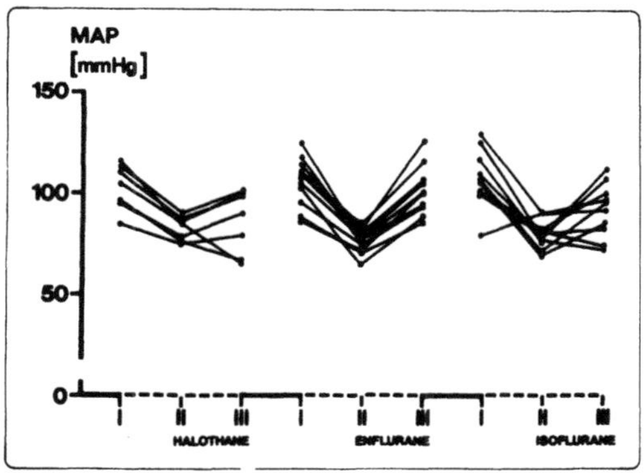

Figure 11 demonstrates that halothane, enflurane and isoflurane-nitrous oxide anaesthesia were associated with a significant decrease in the oxygen consumption of the left ventricle and in myocardial metabolism together with a decrease in myocardial blood flow (fig. 12), all changes being the result of decrased haemodynamic load on the myocardium and a decrease in contractility. Surgical stimulation reversed the effects of the three anaesthetics on myocardial oxygen consumption, metabolism and coronary blood flow, due to an increase in myocardial work. In all groups with the patients at rest, normal coronary blood flow, oxygen and substrate supply and metabolism were maintained and there was no clinical or metabolic evidence of myocardial ischaemia in any patient.

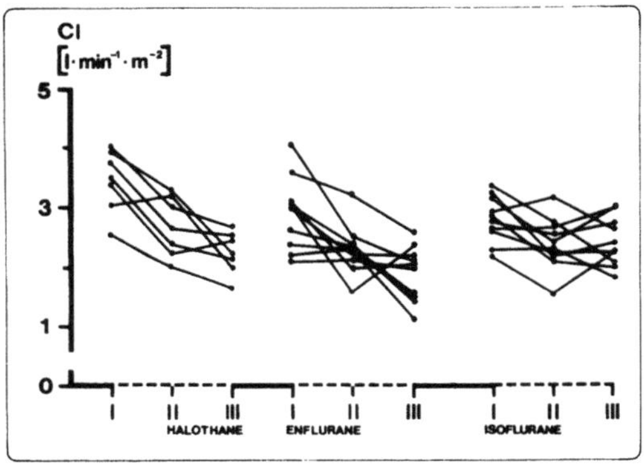

Fig. 9

Fig. 10

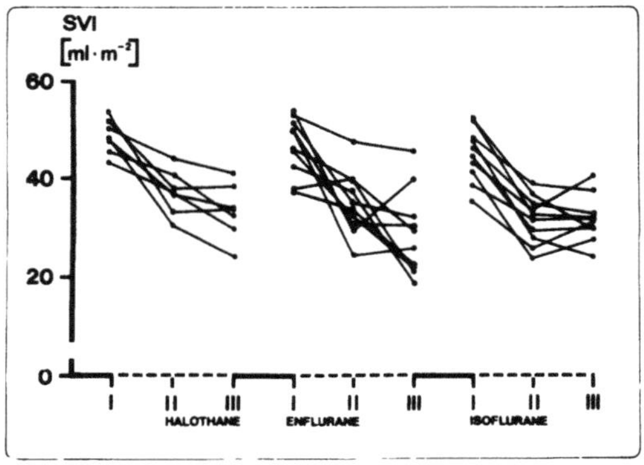

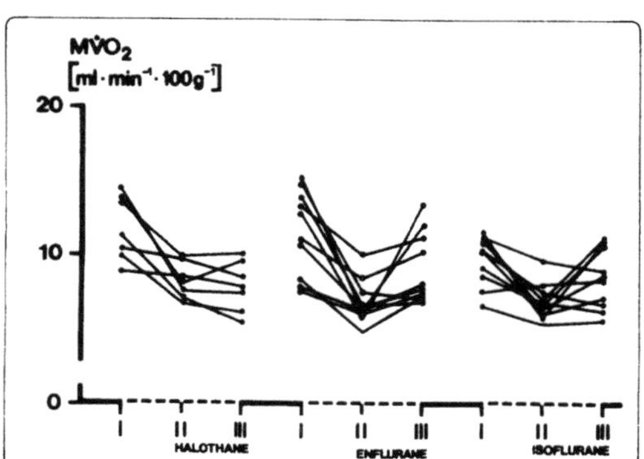

Fig. 11

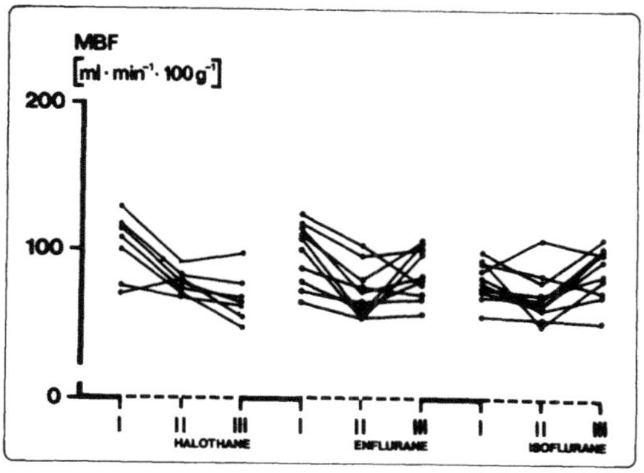

Fig. 12

These findings indicate that poststenotic arteriolar dilatation compensated for the increased resistance in the diseased extramural coronary arteries. After induction of anaesthesia, myocardial metabolism was reduced in all groups to a similar degree, probably due to a net decrease in oxygen demand, while surgical stimulation had the opposite effect, thus indicating, that the myocardial metabolic effects of halothane, enflurane and isoflurane depand on their influence on the haemodynamic determinants of myocardial oxygen consumption and are not induced by a specific interference with biochemical pathways in the myocardium. All three anaesthetics produced some degree of myocardial "luxury perfusion", i.e. myocardial blood flow in excess of demand.
This is evidenced by an increase in the coronary sinus oxygen saturation (fig. 13) together with a decrease in arterial-coronary sinus oxygen content difference and myocardial oxygen consumption and no change in coronary vascular resistance, the effect being more pronounced with isoflurane.

Fig. 13

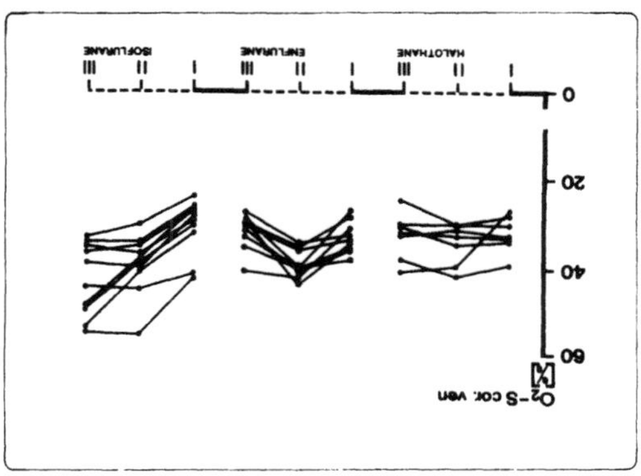

The data indicate that the close coupling of myocardial metabolism and coronary blood flow is impaired by inhalational anaesthetics, probably due to their dilatory actions on the coronary vessels.

Myocardial lactate production (fig. 14) was observed during isoflurane-nitrous oxide anaesthesia in one patient after induction despite a 10% increase in diastolic arterial pressure, with heart rate remaining unchanged. Also, myocardial lactate release did occur in three additional patients of the isoflurane group during sternotomy without abnormal responses in arterial pressure or heart rate. No such effects were observed with halothane and enflurane.

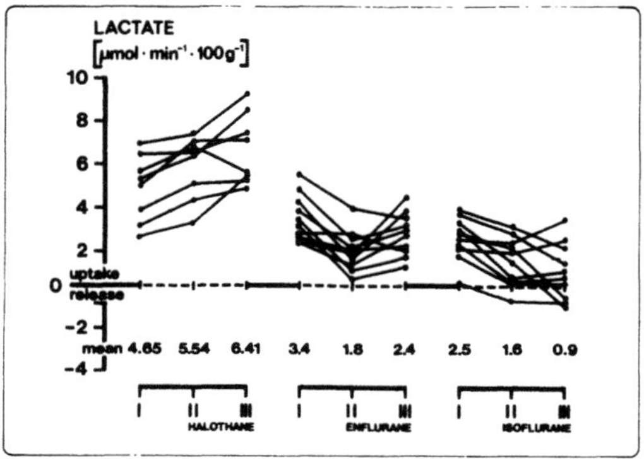

Fig. 14

While there is no doubt that net myocardial lactate production during isoflurane anaesthesia indicates the qualitative presence of myocardial hypoxia, a quantitative relationship between the severity of ischaemia and the amount of lactate production cannot be established from studies of the coronary sinus. It appears from this and the studies of other investigators that myocardial lactate production is not due to a specific effect of isoflurane on metabolic pathway of the myocardium but is rather brought about by haemodynamic changes, that is a decrease in coronary perfusion pressure together with coronary vasodilatation and redistribution of coronary blood flow. Probably these effects of isoflurane on the coronary circulation are of clinical importance in patients with significant coronary artery stenosis and might be produced by any other inhalation anaesthetic with coronary vasodilating and hypotensive properties in these patients.

---

*Supported by the German Research Foundation SFB 89 - Cardiology Göttingen

SEQUENTIAL MYOCARDIAL DEPRESSANT AND NON-DEPRESSANT ANAESTHESIA FOR CORONARY ARTERY SURGERY

G. SETTERGREN

The aim of coronary artery surgery is to eliminate myocardial ischemia distal to critical coronary artery stenoses. This aim is not fulfilled if early graft occlusion occurs. A low graft flow measured during surgery predicts an increased risk of graft occlusion (1-4). Thus it could be of value to study the effect of various anaesthetic regimens on graft blood flow. A "high pressure-high demand" technique would probably be accompanied by a comparatively higher graft flow than a "low pressure-low demand technique".

Before cardiopulmonary bypass (CPB) the situation is different and the aim of the anaesthetic management is easier to define. The important thing is to avoid ischemia, if possible. Some patients come to anaesthesia with angina and ECG-signs of ischemia and in these patients treatment with i.v. nitroglycerin has to be started before the induction of anaesthesia. I.v. nitroglycerin 1 $ug.kg^{-1}.min^{-1}$ has also recently been recommended as a prophylactic treatment during anaesthesa and surgery in patients with ischemic heart disease (5).

It is still a matter of debate which anaesthetic technique will most likely prevent ischemia in te prebypass period, since clearcut signs of ischemia have been demonstrated to occur both with intravenous and inhalational techniques. Apart from the choice of technique a number of things are important, individual titration of dosage, timing in relation to endotracheal intubation and to surgical events and a proper use of vasoactive drugs, most often to reduce afterload but sometimes also to restore vascular tone.

If a combination of i.v. induction followed by inhalational anaesthesia supplemented with an analgesic is used with the intention to obtain a moderate reduction in arterial pressure and to avoid tachycardia, i.e. a moderate "low pressure-low demand" state, I believe that the risk of ischemia would be less than with techniques resulting in "high pressure -high demand" situations. It would not be an easy task, however, to prove the correctness of such a statement. The mortality in connection with coronary artery surgery is low and so is the frequency of periooperative myocardial infarction. This implies that large series have to be compared. Additional problems are the influence of surgery on the complications and the risk of bias in those conducting the anaesthetics in a controlled, randomized study.

When waiting for surgery patients with coronary artery stenoses are advised to restrict their physical activity and to avoid situations provoking angina in order to diminish the risk of myocardial infarction. After surgery if revascularization has been successful, this attitude is changed and many patients are introduced to training programs with the aim that they should regain a more normal working capacity.

The things mentioned above were the background for the concept of sequential myocardial depressant and non-depressant anaesthesia for coronary artery surgery.

In a study published recently (6) the hemodynamic effects of a technique based on halothane before cardiopulmonary bypass followed by i.v. anaesthesia with fentnayl, droperidol and diazepam after CPB were studied. In the first 7 patients bradycardia during rewarming and reperfusion was observed. In these patients the administration of halothane had been stopped immediately before CPB. A residual effect of halothane was suspected and consequently halothane was discontinued 10-15 minutes before CPB in the following 7 patients. In this latter group the desired hemodynamic effect was most clearly observed. Left ventricular power index (LVPI) i.e. the work per unit time of the left ventricle was calculated since this parameter probably is correlated to graft blood flow. The control value of LVPI in the awak premedicated patient with coronary artery disease is 0.69 $W.m^{-2}$ (S.D. 0.24) in our department. Mean LVPI was 0.35-0.52 $W.m^{-2}$ before CPB and increased significantly to 0.62-0.76 $W.m^{-2}$ in the postbypass period. It is reasonable to assume that the normalization of LVPI promoted a high graft blood flow compared to a situlation with a reduced LVPI, should the inhalational anaesthesia have been continued. The relation between filling pressure (measured as pulmonary artery diastolic pressure) and left ventricular stroke work index tended to be different in the prebypass period compared to postbypass indicating a moderatly depressed left ventricular function in the prebypass period and a more normal function curve after bypass.

A combination of a reduced work load and a maintained graft flow would, however, be ideal in the postbypass period. The effect of nitrous oxide on coronary graft blood flow in the period immediately after CPB has recently been studied (7). N_2O caused a reversible reduction of myocardial pressure work and contractility in combination with an unchanged graft flow. Nitrous oxide is, however, potentially dangerous in situations with air embolization. Several moments in coronary artery surgery, such as cannulation of the aorta, suturing of the proximal anastomoses, insertion of a left ventricular vent or a left atrial catheter, carry a certain risk of air embolization to the systemic circulation. Although these complications are rare, they may be unnoticed during surgery and are first suspected in the postoperative period. Thus the use of nitrous oxide in the post-bypass period is controversial.

In later studies from our groups the effect of various other agents that reduce systemic arterial pressure in the period after CPB, have been investigated. Isoflurane had been shown to reduce cardiac work without a concomitant decrease in coronary sinus blood flow both experimentally in dogs (8) and in unpremedicated man(9). When tested in the post-bypass period, however, isoflurane caused a decrease in graft flow by 23% when LVPI was reduced from 0.75 to 0.44 $W.m^{-2}$ (10). In contrast, adenosine in continuous infusion 40 $ug.kg^{-1}.min^{-1}$ caused a reversible increase in graft flow by 80% while LVPI remained unchanged at 0.53 $W.m^{-2}$ due to a reduced arterial pressure balanced by an increased stroke volume (11).

To conclude: Anaesthetic techniques used for coronary artery surgery should be evaluated not only in relation to the porblems of ischemia but also with respect to their effect on bypass graft flow. Sequential myocardial depressant and non-depressant anaesthesia promoted graft flow by normalization of the work load of the heart already in the post-bypass period during surgery. With a continuous infusion of adenosine in a low dose graft flow was increased concomitant with an unchanged or reduced cardiac work. These techniques need further evaluation.

REFERENCES

1. Grondin GM, Lepage G, Castonguay Y, Meere C, Grondin P: Aortocoronary venous bypass grafts: Initial blood flow through the graft and early postoperative patency. Circulation 1979: 42: Suppl 3: 106-110.
2. Campeau L, Crochet D, Lésperance J, Bourassa MG, Gronding GM: Postoperative changes in aortocoroanry saphenous vein grafts revisited: Angiographic studies at two weeks and at one year in two series of consecutive patients. Circulation 1975: 52: 269-277.
3. Roth JA, Cuningnan RA, Brown BG, Gocka G, Carey JS: Factors influencing patency of saphenous vein grafts, Ann Thorac Surg 1979: 28: 176-182.
4. Björk VO, Ekeström S, Henze A, Ivert T, Landou C: Early and late patency of coronary vein grafts. Scand J Thor Cardiovasc Surg 1981: 15: 11-21.
5. Coriat P, Daloz M, Bousseau D, Fusciardi J, Echter E, Viars P: Prevention of intraoperative myocardial ischemia during noncardiac surgery with intravenous nitroglycerin, Anesthesiology 1984: 61: 193-196.
6. Settergren G, ÖHqvist G, Ekeström S: Sequential myocardial depressant and non-depressant anaesthesia for coronary artery surgery. Acta Anaesthsiol Scand 1985: 29: 26-31.
7. Lilleaasen P, Semb B, Lindberg H, Hatteland K, Ottesen S, Simonsen S: Haemodynamic changes with the administration of nitrous oxide during coronary artery surgery. Acta Anaesthesiol Scand 1981: 25: 533-537.
8. Tarnow J, Eberlein HJ, Oser G: Hämodynamik, Myokardkontraktilität, Ventrikelvolumina und Sauerstoffversorgerung des Herzens unter verschiedenen Inhalationsanestetika. Anaesthesist 1977: 26: 220-230.
9. Reiz S, Bålfors E, Bredgaard-Sörensen MS, Ariola Jr S, Friedman A, Truedsson H: Isoflurane - a powerful coronary vasodilator in patients with coronary artery disease. Anesthesiology 1983: 59: 91-97.
10. Öhqvist G, Settergren G, Ekeström S, Brodin LÅ: The influence of isoflurane on blood flow in coronary bypass grafts. Acta Anaesthesiol Scand. Accepted for publication.
11. Torssell L, Sollevi A, Ekeström S, Öhqvist G: Unpublished data.

CONTINUOUS ARTERIAL pH-MONITORING FOLLOWING CORONARY ARTERY BYPASS SURGERY.

Peter J.A. van der Starre, M.D., Joukje E. Harinck-de Weerd, M.D.,
Siep J. Schepel, M.S.

INTRODUCTION

In the early postoperative period following coronary artery bypass surgery, quick changes can occur in blood gases and electrolytes (1). Usually the patients are hypothermic, when they arrive in the intensive care unit and during the first 6 to 8 hours the temperature rises peripherally as well as centrally. Due to haemodilution the haematocrit is generally low, between 25 and 28% (2), and mainly due to diuresis, increases to 30 to 32% in the same period. Hypertension develops in 30 to 60% of the patients, treated with anti-hypertensive agents, mainly consisting of vasodilating agents (3,7). When the patients wake up, and are still unable to breath on their own, they are sedated by using benzodiazepines (midazolam). Shivering is treated by the use of muscle relaxants in a low dose, but when the patient is well awake and able to respond on command, weaning off ventilation is started. To achieve this synchronized intermittent mandatory ventilation (SIMV) technique is applied, and when blood gases are within acceptable limits the patient is extubated. Usually this happens between 6 to 10 hours postoperatively (1).
If in this postoperative period a patient develops acidosis, strong influences can occur on for example myocardial contractility, regional bloodflow, and on the effectiveness of the pharmacological treatment, because of changes in protein-binding, receptor-binding, renal excretion and metabolism (4,5).
Usually these changes are followed in the laboratory tests intermittently, but for above mentioned reasons it can be interesting to follow changes in the pH continuously.

MATERIALS AND METHODS

A 7 French double lumen catheter was inserted in the early postoperative period in the I.C.U. in 15 patients, using the femoral artery as the introduction site. Beforehand APTT and PTT were analysed, and confirmed to be with normal limits. The catheter was introduced through a Seldinger technique through an introducer set, which was left in place. In the tip of the catheter an ISFET chip (ISFET = ion selective field effect transistor) is incorporated in the catheter with a smooth surface to prevent thrombogenesis. The clinical advantages of a semi-conducter chip are mainly the short response time and the low output impedance. The catheter is not heparinized (6,8).
The catheter is connected with a monitor, which contains a microprocessor especially designed for signal conversion and temperature correction. After a stabilization period of about 15 minutes the catheter is calibrated against a sample analysis, using an ABL-blood gas analyser.

RESULTS

Figure 1. After calibration it appeared that the intermittent pH sampling and the continuous pH monitoring correlated well during a 12 hour study period in the I.C.U. The pH monitor follows changes in pH accurately, which gave the opportunity to study the events during this period more in detail.

pH monitoring in an ICU patient over 12 hours

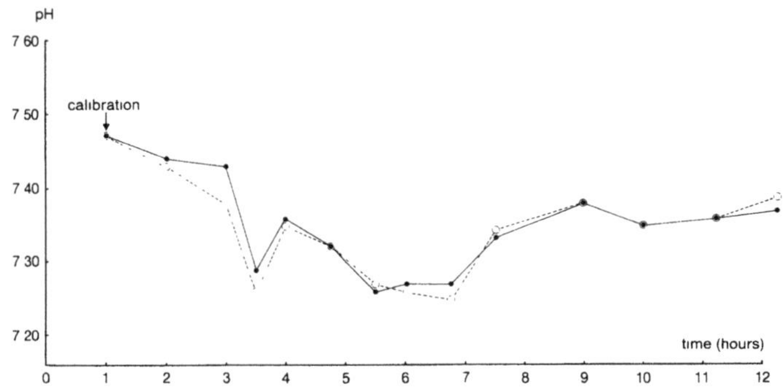

Figure 2. Changes in minute volume, like for example an increase from 8.5 to 9.5 litres per minute are followed accurately by the pH monitor, indicating an increase in pH to about 7.4 in a period of about 10 minutes.

Change in MV ($8\frac{1}{2} \rightarrow 9\frac{1}{2}$ l/min)

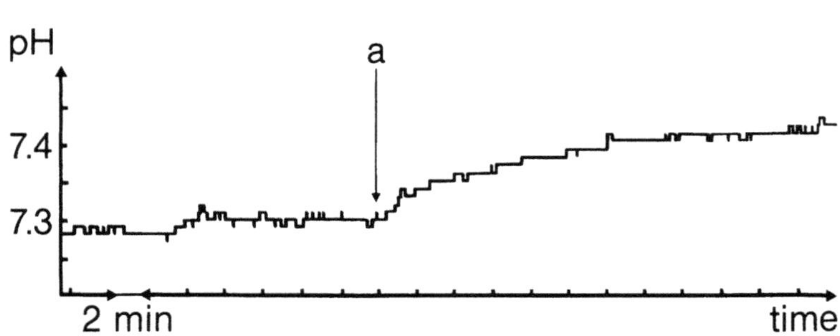

00876 B18(1)-5220

Figure 3. Respiratory monitoring intra- and postoperatively has been developed in the last 10 years in the direction of capnography. In this study a continuous end-tidal CO_2 monitoring and a continuous pH monitoring were compared in view of the response to changes in minute volume. A 30 seconds ventilator stand-still is depicted, indicating that the continuous pH monitoring reveals substantial changes with respect to the acid base balance, while the end-tidal CO_2 response is minimal. It is an example of the very short response time of the ISFET chip.

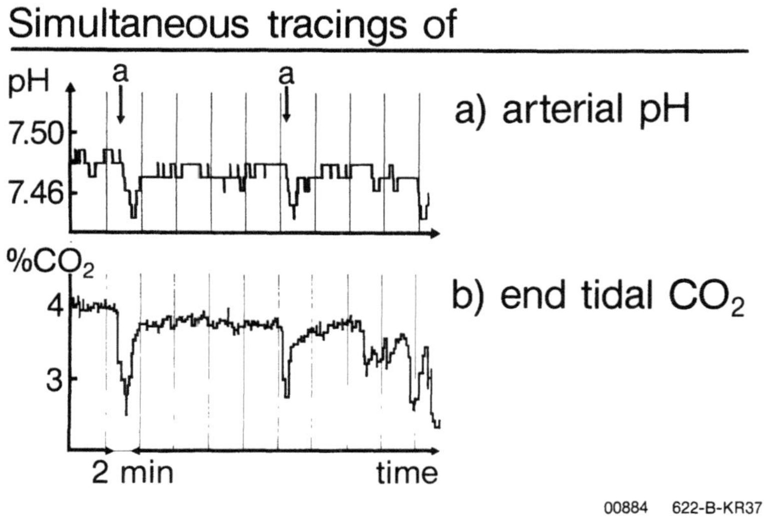

Figure 4 and figure 5. When the patient is on the ventilator and wakes up, and the assumption is made that he should be able to breath on his own, weaning is started using a SIMV method.
In this study two patterns could be detected with respect to this weaning procedure:

Figure 4. Indicates pattern 1, which means that at the first attempts to start weaning, pH decreases substantially, and remains at a lower level all through the weaning procedure.

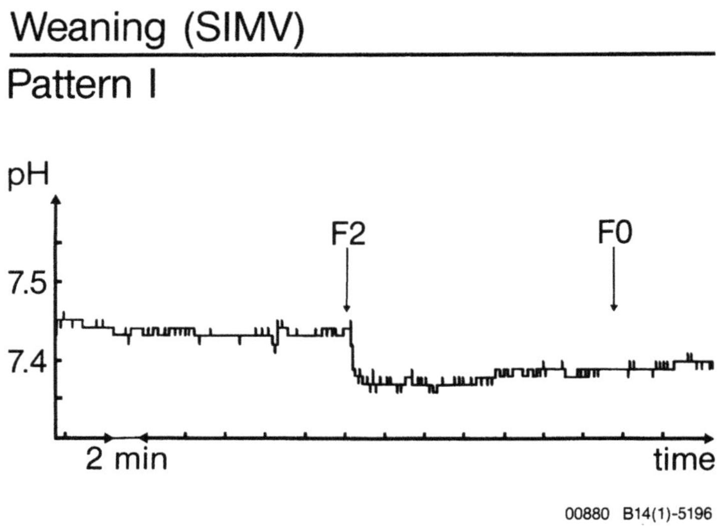

Figure 5. Indicates another pattern, in which this lower level of pH is recorded only when the patient is breathing completely on his own (FO).

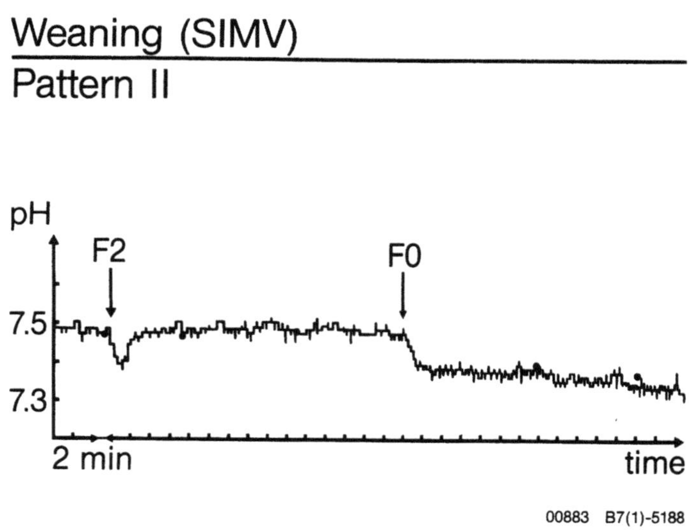

Figure 6. Starting of weaning does not always follow a smooth pattern. Regaining of consciousness can go parallel with panicking of the patient, in which a start of weaning procedure can lead to severe acidosis. Usually this period causes hypertension, coughing, tachycardia. The ventilator has to be reset on controlled ventilation.

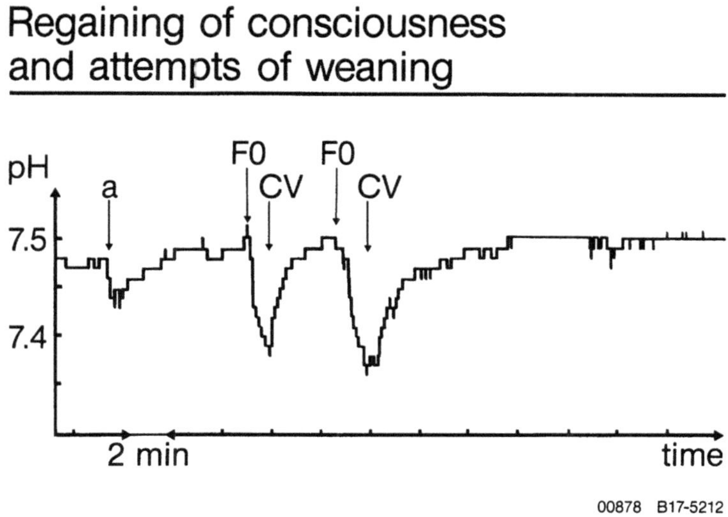

Figure 7. Successful verbal support can improve the patient's effort when weaning is started.
In period a. the patient's efforts were insufficient to start SIMV, because he was desorientated. In period b. verbal support from the assisting nurse enabled the patient to start the SIMV procedure.

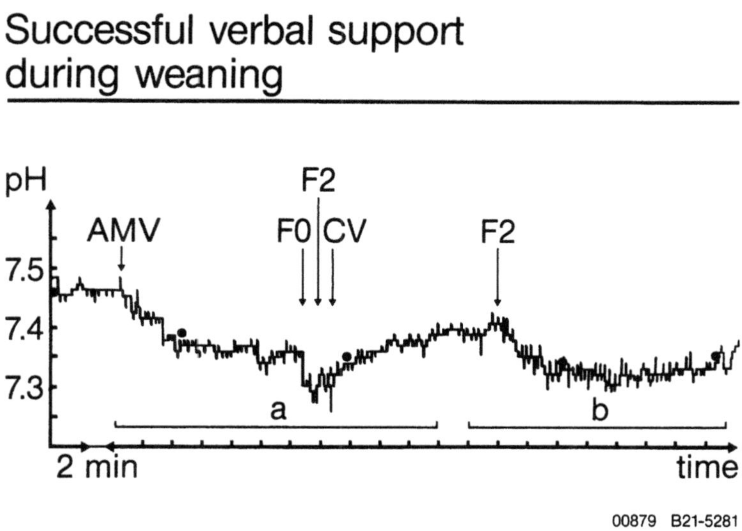

Figure 8. When the patient wakes up, or when bronchial suction is applied coughing can lead to substantial changes in pH, from alcalosis to acidosis.

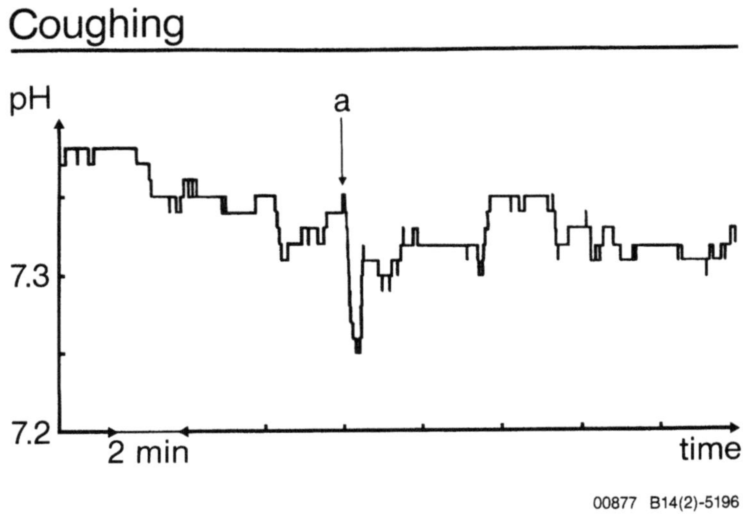

Figure 9. Shows the effect of the inhalation of bronchodilating agents as is usually applied in patients with COPD. The recording shows that there was no influence of these agents on the pH pattern during a spontaneously breathing patient.

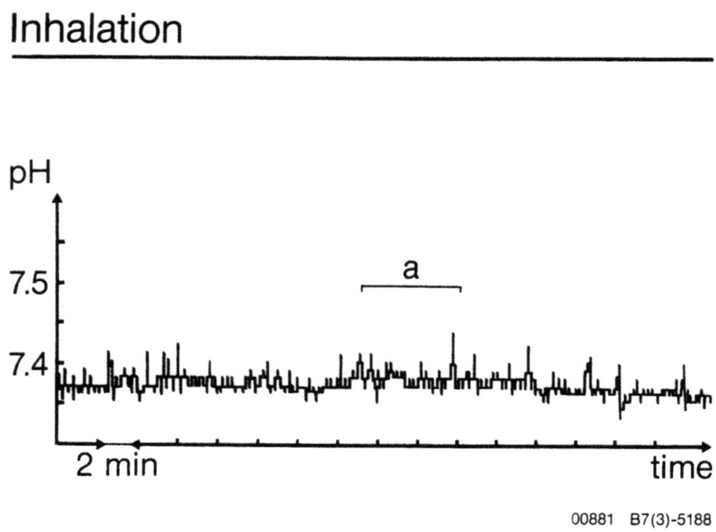

Figure 10. When the SIMV procedure has been successful, and the patient is extubated, after assessing that the blood gases were within normal limits, a pattern develops of own respiration. This pattern reveals that during breathing continuous changes in a very short response time occur in a cyclic way.

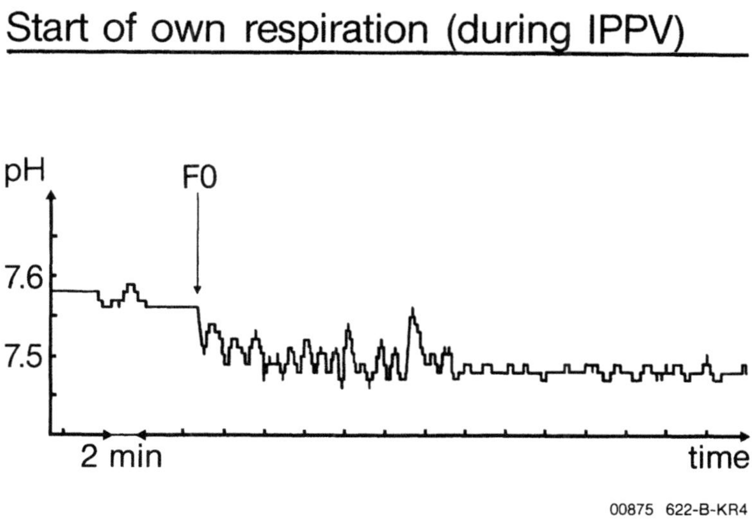

DISCUSSION

Changes in pH and electrolytes in the early postoperative period in patients following major surgery can lead to changes in for example myocardial contractility, regional blood flow and the efficacy of pharmacological treatment (4,5). In the study group, consisting of patients who were operated for coronary artery disease, the pH changes were monitored by a continuous recording, using an invasive pH monitoring technique (6,8). Since pH is determined in this setting mainly by changes in the pCO_2, the ventilatory pattern of a patient on a mechanical ventilator, followed by a SIMV-procedure, could be monitored in detail. It was obvious that two patterns of weaning could be detected, and especially procedures like coughing and bronchial suction can have strong influences on the pH, leading to severe acidosis in a short time. It is not surprising that reports have been made with respect to arrythmias, even leading to ventricular fibrillation and low cardiac output syndrome, in a period of bronchial suction.

A third interesting observation was that during spontaneous breathing, the ISFET chip, with a very short response time, showed that cyclic changes occur in pH, revealing cyclic changes in pCO_2.

It is especially interesting to follow the ventilatory pattern following cardiopulmonary bypass, because earlier reports have shown that there is an increase in lung water following these procedures, leading to an increase in shunt fraction and a decrease in FRC (9,10).

In conclusion this study showed that there appeared to be a good correlation between the continuous measurements of pH and the intermittent sample analysis of the blood gases, there was a good stability of the pH-monitoring, the response to changes in the pH due to changes in the ventilatory pattern was fast, and the continuous monitoring of pH revealed important clinical phenomena during the study period. A disadvantage of the technique was, that the femoral artery had te be cannulated because of the size of the catheter, which for routine application is still too large. Eventually one might assume that the continuous monitoring of pH, giving opportunity to titrate changes in pH using for example bicarbonate or by changing a ventilatory pattern, opens a new research with respect to pharmacological and fysiological studies.

REFERENCES

1. Hinds CJ. Current management of patients after cardiopulmonary bypass Anaesthesia 1982;37:170-191
2. Sladen RN. Temperature changes and ventilation after hypothermic cardiopulmonary bypass.
3. Estafanous FG, Tarizi RC. Systemic arterial hypertension associated with cardiac surgery. Am. J. Cardiol. 1980;46:685-704
4. Cingolani HE, Faulkuer SL, Mattiazzi AR, et al. Depression of human myocardial contractility with respiratory and metabolic acidosis. Surgery 1975;77:427-432
5. Clowes GHA, Sabga GA, Komitaxis A, et al. Effects of acidosis on cardiovascular function in sugical patients. Ann. of Surg. 1961;154:524-555
6. Schepel SJ, de Rooij NF, Koning G, et al. In vivo experiments with a pH-ISFET electrode. Med. Biol. Comput 1984;22:6-11
7. Anjon Lindskog E, Broman L, Holmgren A. Effects of nitroglycerin on central haemodynamics and V_a/Q distribution early after coronary artery bypass surgery. Acta. An. Scand. 1982;26:489-497
8. Bergveld P. Development, operation and application of the ion selective field effect transistor as a tool physiology. IEEE Trans 1972; 19:342-351
9. Ali J, Weisel RD, Layng AB, et al. Consequences of postoperative alterations in respiratory mechanics. A. J. Surg. 1974;128:376-382
10. Anyaunwu E, Dittrich H, Gieseking R, Enders HJ. Ultrastructural changes in the lumen lung following cardiopulmonary bypass. Basic Res. Cardiol. 1982;77:309-322

THE MANAGEMENT OF CARDIAC EMERGENCIES - CARDIAC TAMPONADE

SIMON DE LANGE

INTRODUCTION

Cardiac tamponade is a life-threatening complication occuring after thoracic trauma or cardiac surgery. Blood, other fluids or even air may accumulate in the pericardial cavity. A rise of intrapericardial pressure ensues which can severely impede cardiac action. The acuity of onset of symptoms depends on the rate of fluid accumulation. Complete cardiac collapse may occur within seconds or symptoms may take weeks to develop; decompression is the only cure.

The role of the anesthesiologist is that of providing supportive therapy, analgesia, and when indicated, safe anaesthesia until decompression is accomplished.

Classification and Aetiology

ACUTE
- after thoracic trauma (blunt or penetrating injury)
- folowing open heart surgery
- iatrogenic (catheterisation pacing wires, pericardiocentesis)

DELAYED
- 7 days to three months after cardiac surgery or trauma

MEDICAL CAUSES
- neoplasm
- uraemia
- ideopathic

A British survey revealed that less than half the casulaties with penetrating cardiac injury died before reaching hospital; those alive on admission had a better than 90% survival rate (1). In studies from more violent areas of the world, cardiac tamponade was found in the majority of patients undergoing surgery for penetrating stab or gunshot wounds of the heart. But, those patients with tamponade had a 12-16% mortality rate (2.3). Thus, cardiac tamponade may prolong survival by delaying exsanguination but may itself cause cardiovascular collapse. Some centres report that 76% of all thoracic trauma cases have associated blunt cardiac injury (4). Presumably these are situated in areas where the use of seat belts is not compulsory. Cardiac tamponade can develop after non-penetrating trauma and should not be overlooked in these patients.

Following open heart surgery the overall incidence of cardiac tamponade is 3-6%; leaving the anterior pericardium open does not preclude its development (5). In the immediate post-operative period large blood clots throughout the pericardial cavity may cause compression in spite of freely running drains. Slower accumulation of fluid can result in a confined posterior or anterior pericardial effusion which may cause tamponade of an individual cardiac chamber (6-7).

Incautious postoperative removal of indwelling atrial lines or external pacing wires may result in sudden collapse of the patient due to tamponade. A rare complication of central venous cannulation is perforation of the heart or intrapericardial vessels. The onset of tamponade symptoms is often insiduous and the mortality rate is high (78-95%), mainly due to late recognition of the problem (8). Needle puncture of the heart may occur during pericardiocentesis for acute tamponade and precipitate collapse; this procedure is not recommended in acute cases (1-3).

Delayed cardiac tamponade is defined as one that manifests itself one or more weeks after cardiac surgery. It is considered to be a complication of anticoagulant therapy or postpericardiotomy syndrome (5, 6, 9, 10). The pericardium can slowly stretch over a period of several weeks so that volumes of over 2 litres of serous or sanguinous fluid can be tolerated (6, 9). Although a rare complication (1.3-2.2%), it is often fatal because it is not promptly recognized as a cause of postoperative low output syndrome (6, 7, 9, 10).

Patients with neoplastic disease or uraemia may accumulate large compressing pericardial effusions. The management of these medical patients, as well as patients with delayed cardiac tamponade, is different to those with acute traumatic or post-operative tamponade in that they usually undergo decompression by needle pericardiocentesis and thus are not seen by the anaesthesiologist.

Pathophysiology

The compliance of the pericardium is low so that rapid expansion of the pericardial fluid from the normal 30-50 ml to 150-200 ml can profoundly affect cardiac function. However, the pericardium slowly regains its original configuration so that removal of only 50 ml of blood can dramatically improve haemodynamic status (5).

Increasing intrapericardial pressure has its initial major effect on the low-pressure heart chambers and vessels (11,12). Right atrial collapse occurs early in the morbid process; right ventricular collapse appears later by which time cardiac output is depressed but systemic blood pressure is maintained. This is known as the compensated phase: the catecholamine-mediated stress response has increased myocardial contractility and heart rate; arterial vasoconstriction and venoconstriction also assist in elevating the venous pressure in order to maintain cardiac filling.

Eventually cardiovascular collapse occurs due to inadequate filling of the ventricle, even though the pump function of the left ventricle may be well preserved in patients without myocardial or valvular disease (13). Cardiac tamponade also reduces coronary perfusion, not only by the extrinsic pressure effect which decreases the endocardial to epicardial blood flow ratio but also by the accompanying tachycardia (14). Patients with myocardial disease poorly tolerate tamponade: impaired coronary perfusion rapidly causes myocardial ischaemia which further decreases myocardial contractility and output. A viscious circle is set up which quickly progresses to haemodynamic collapse or the decompensated phase (15).

Signs

Increasing venous pressure
Distant heart sound
Decreasing arterial pressure
Pulses paradoxus
Distended neck veins (Kussmaul's sign)
Tachycardia
Pallor

Following acute penetrating cardiac trauma these signs have proved useful in confirming the diagnosis except pulsus paradoxus (decrease of systolic blood pressure by 10-20 mmHg during inspiration) which was rarely observed (2-3). Postoperatively these signs of cardiac tamponade are not so apparent: heart sounds may have normal intensity if the pericardium has been left open, increased venous pressure and tachycardia may have other causes and raised venous pressure may only be demonstrable after hypovolaemia has been corrected. Pulsus paradoxus, if observed, may not be diagnostic since it occurs quite often in mechanically ventilated patients especially if they are also hypovolaemic (1, 5, 15).

Diagnostic Aids

Serial chest films showing progressive enlargement of the cardiopericardial shadow clearly confirm suspicion of tamponade. In contrast, unless changes are dramatic, portable chest films may be unreliable in assisting diagnosis after penetrating cardiac trauma or after cardiac surgery (2, 3, 15).

ECG changes are usually non-specific. Ventricular electrical alternans is sometimes observed and, if marked, stongly indicates tamponade (16). Idioventricular rhythms associated with cardiac injury are not infrequently seen and have a sinister prognosis (3).

The echocardiogram can identify large pericardial effusions but may not clearly illustrate blood clots or relatively small posterior pericardial effusions which may cause compression in the immediate postoperative period (5, 15). The main diagnostic value of echocardiography is in observing cardiac action since right atrial and right ventricular collapse are sensitive and accurate markers of cardiac tamponade (12, 17).

Haemodynamic monitoring, especially by way of a pulmonary artery catheter, is the most valuable method of establishing a diagnosis. Restriction of cardiac filling not only results in elevation of right-sided pressure but also leads to their close approximation. Right atrial, right ventricular, pulmonary artery diastolic and pulmonary capillary wedge pressures become almost identical and form a "pressure plateau" (5, 15). When this sign is combined with decreasing cardiac output it strongly suggests cardiac tamponade.

Differential diagnosis

Postoperatively, acute right ventricular infarction may simulate cardiac tamponade, but in the majority of patients there is ECG evidence of infarction. In addition, right ventricular end diastolic pressure is disproportionally elevated.

Massive pulmonary embolism will cause rapid elevation of the right atrial and right ventricular pressure but the pulmonary artery capillary wedge pressure will be relatively normal (5, 15).

Air trapped in the pericardial cavity is increasingly being recognized as a cause of cardiac compression. Tension pneumopericardium is most frequently seen in penetrating cardiac trauma patients (where massive air embolism is an added hazard) and in neonates on positive pressure ventilation (2, 18). It has a sinister prognosis with a mortality rate of 56%. Chest radiographs clearly indicate the diagnosis.

Supportive therapy

In acute tamponade the only therapy is decompression. If the diagnosis is not yet definite or time is required before elective surgery supportive therapy can prolong survival.

1) Correct hypovolaemia and optimize filling pressures

A fluid challenge should be tried to exclude hypovolaemia especially in acute traumatic tamponade. Thereafter central venous pressure can be raised to 20 mmHg or higher which may improve cardiac filling by elevating intracardial pressure above intrapericardial but, it may exacerbate myocardial ischaemia (15, 16, 19).

2) Positive inotropic agents (augmentation of stress response)

Dopamine or isoprenaline have been shown to increase cardiac output during acute tamponade (14-16, 20). Their use is generally considered to be beneficial but they increase myocardial work and tachycardia which may cause myocardial ischaemia.

3) Vasodilators

Vasodilating drugs together with fluid expansion have been recommended as emergency therapy in experimental tamponade. However, in non-hypovolaemic patients with acute medical tamponade, fluid expansion and nitroprusside infusion were found to be of little haemodynamic benefit (19). In hypovolaemic patients afterload reduction with nitroprusside would seem to be perilous therapy. Nitroglycerine is also contraindicated because its principle effect is reduction of preload.

4) Pericardiocentesis

Therapeutic or diagnostic periocardicentesis is not recommended in acute tamponade after trauma or cardiac surgery since the exploratory needle may puncture the atria or ventricles and exacerbate the morbid process (1-3). Furthermore, the tap may be negative in spite of large blood clots or a compressing posterior pericardial effusion. If employed as a temporizing measure the needle should be used as an exploring ECG electrode to avoid inadvertant myocardial damage (19).

SURGICAL APPROACH

Median sternotomy is becoming the favoured surgical approach for elective decompression after cardiac trauma as it allows optimum inspection of the intrapericardial structures (2-3). Following cardiac surgery the sternal wound can be quickly reopened by cutting the sternal wires, if need be in the intensive care unit.

Left anterior lateral thoracotomy provides rapid access as an emergency procedure in the moribund trauma patient (1-3).

Subxiphoid pericardial window is an initial elective approach which allows decompression but not adequate inspection of the heart and great vessels after surgery or trauma (21).

Anaesthetic Essentials

MAINTAIN - venous filling pressure
- tachycardia
- vasoconstriction

AVOID - myocardial depression
- sudden vasodilatation
- intermittant positive pressure ventilation (IPPV)

All currently used volatile inhalational agents and most intravenous anaesthetic agents depress myocardial contractility and are peripheral vasodilators so that their injudicious use will cause haemodynamic collapse in tamponading patients (16, 21). Preoperative sedation, although humane, may similarly precipitate decompensation. Narcotic analgesics blunt the patients stress response when he really needs additional sympathomimetic support and should be used with extreme caution. Ketamine centrally stimulates the release of endogenous catecholamines as well as providing dissociative anaesthesia. It is recommended as an intravenous induction agent and for maintaining anaesthesia until tamponade has been released (15, 16).

Various authors have advised against IPPV as it furthur decreases cardiac output in the presence of cardiac tamponade (16, 21, 22). It appears that positive pressure changes in the pleural cavity are faithfully transmitted to the compressing pericardial fluid (22). However, in practice many patients with acute traumatic tamponade may have been intubated and ventilated as part of the resuscitative procedure. Furthermore, patients after open heart surgery are usually mechanically ventilated. In these cases experimental work suggests that IPPV may be maintained provided positive end expiratory pressure and slow frequency ventilation is avoided (20).

Anaesthetic Techniques

Premedication is minimized or omitted.

Local anaesthetic infiltration

A subxiphoid subpericardial window is made using less than 30 ml 1% lidocaine for infiltration anaesthesia (21). A recent median sternotomy facilitates reopening of the lower end of the sternum using local anaesthesia. These techniques are safe but unpleasant for the patient.

Ketamine 2.5 $mg.kg^{-1}$ and local anaesthetic infiltration

There is dissociative anaesthesia and spontaneous ventilation can be maintained but unless already intubated the airway may not be secure in a critically ill patient. To avoid this problem, Möller and coworkers have suggested awake endotracheal intubation using topical anaesthesia (22). This procedure is both traumatic and time consuming unless performed by an expert.

Ketamine 1-2 $mg.kg^{-1}$ suxamethonium, endotracheal intubation

Following preoxygenation and atropine IV, a ketamine-suxamethonium sequence allows rapid endotracheal intubation. Spontaneous ventilation can resume, if deemed necessary. Maintenance of anaesthesia is with ketamine (0,5-1,0 $mg.kg^{-1}$ bolus doses) or, if the haemodynamic status is adequate, carefully titrated nitrous oxide (25-50%).

After decompression and restoration of cardiovascular stability any favoured general anaesthesia technique may safely be employed if furthur intrapericardial exploration is necessary (15, 16, 21).

CONCLUSION

Knowledge of the pathophysiology of acute cardiac tamponade helps the anaesthesiologist to recognize the clinical signs and to interpret the monitoring information of this potentially lethal complication. Early awareness and suspicion of the possibility of tamponade may reduce morbidity and mortality.

Supportive therapy may gain time to prepare for elective surgery but may also increase myocardial ischaemia.

Anaesthesia does not improve the haemodynamic status of the patient only decompression provides dramatic improvement.

REFERENCES

1. Reece IJ, Davidson KG: Emergency surgery for stab wounds to the heart. Ann R Coll Surg Engl 65: 304-307, 1983.
2. Demetriades D: Cardiac penetrating injuries: personal experience of 45 cases. Br J Surg 71: 95-97, 1984.
3. Marshall WG, Bell JL, Kouchoukos NT: Penetrating cardiac trauma. J Trauma 24: 147-149, 1984.
4. Griffith GL, Zeok JV, Mattingly WT, Todd EP: Right atrial rupture due to blunt chest trauma. South Med J 77: 715-716, 1984.
5. Weeks KR, Chatterjee K, Block S, Matloff JM, Swan HJC: Bedside hemodynamic monitoring. J Thorac Cardiovasc Surg 71: 250-252, 1976.
6. Borkon AM, Schaff HV, Gardner TJ, Merrill WH, Brawley RK, Donahoo JS, Watkins L, Weiss JL, Gott VL: Diagnosis and management of postoperative pericardial effusions and late cardiac tamponade following open-heart surgery. Ann Thorac Surg 31: 512-519, 1980.
7. Jones MR, Vine DL, Attas M, Todd EP: Late isolated ventricular tamponade. J Thorac Cardiovasc Surg 77: 142-146, 1979.
8. Maschke SP, Rogove HJ: Cardiac tamponade associated with a multilumen central venous catheter. Crit Care Med 12: 611-613, 1984.
9. Bortolotti U, Livi U, Frugoni C, de Mozzi P, Mazzucco A, Valfrè C, Gallucci V: Delayed cardiac tamponade following open heart surgery: analysis of 12 patients. Thorac Cardiovasc Surgeon 29: 233-236, 1981.
10. Merrill W, Donahoo JS, Brawley RK, Taylor D: Late cardiac tamponade: a potentially lethal complication of open-heart surgery. J Thorac Cardiovasc Surg 72: 929-932, 1976.
11. Fowler NO, Gabel M: The hemodynamic effects of cardiac tamponade: mainly the result of atrial not ventricular compression. Circulation 71: 154-157, 1985.
12. Singh S, Wann LS, Schuchard GH, Klopfenstein HS, Leingruber PP, Keelan MH, Brooks HL: Right ventricular and right atrial collapse in patients with cardiac tamponade - a combined echocardigraphic and hemodynamic study. Circulation 70: 966-971, 1984.
13. Grose R, Greenberg M, Steingart R, Cohen MV: Left ventricular volume and function during relief of cardiac tamponade in man. Circulation 66: 149-155, 1982.
14. Martins JB, Manuel WJ, Marcus ML, Kerber RE: Comparative effects of catecholamines in cardiac tamponade: experimental and clinical studies. Am J Cardiol 46: 59-66, 1980.
15. Sladen RN: Management of the adult cardiac patient in the intensive care unit. In: Ream AK, Fogdall RP (eds). Acute cardiovascular management. JB Lippincott Company, Philadelphia, pp 520-524, 1982.
16. Kaplan JA, Bland JW, Dunbar W: The perioperative management of pericardial tamponade. South Med J 69: 417-419, 1976.
17. Gillam LD, Guyer D, Gibson TC, King ME, Marshall J, Weyman AE: Hemodynamic compression of the right atrium: a new echocardiographic sign of cardiac tamponade. Circulation 68: 294-301, 1983.
18. Cummings RG, Wesly RLR, Adams DH, Lowe JE: Pneumopericardium resulting in cardiac tamponade. Ann Thorac Surg 37: 511-518, 1984.
19. Kerber RE, Gascho JA, Litchfiled R, Wolfson P, Ott D, Pandian NG: Hemodynamic effects of volume expansion and nitroprusside compared to pericardiocentesis in patients with acute cardiac tamponade. N Engl J Med 307: 929-931, 1982.
20. Mattila I, Takkunen O, Harjula A, Mattila S, Merikallio E: Cardiac tamponade and different modes of artificial ventilation. Acta Anaesthesiol Scand 28: 236-240, 1984.

21. Stanley TH, Weidauer HE: Anesthesia for the patient with cardiac tamponade. Anesth Analg 52: 110-114, 1973.
22. Möller CT, Schoonbee CG, Rosendorff C: Haemodynamics of cardiac tamponade during various modes of ventilation. Br J Anaesth 51: 409-414, 1979.

LEAKING PROSTHETIC VALVES

J.G. BOVILL

Prosthetic valve reoperations represent a small, but increasing, percentage of all valvular replacement surgery. There are many reasons why a prosthetic valve will need replacement, including wear and tear of the mechanical structures, primary fabric failure or disruption of function due to thrombus formation or endocarditis. In the immediate postoperative phase valve function may be disrupted by suture failure with perivalvular leakage, or intervention of tissue or suture material in the valve mechanism leading to acute incompetence. The newer porcine heterografts are not immune to these problems. The popularity of this type of prosthetic valve has increased steadily from the mid-1970s and, with an assumed durability of 10-12 years, we can expect to see an increasing incidence of reoperations for heterograft failure in the mid- and late-1980s. Modern heterografts are treated with glutaraldehyde, that is more effective than the previously used formalin in decreasing antigenicity but does not completely eliminate it. The remaining weak antigenic stimulus, usually due to residual glycoproteins, results in an inflammatory lymphocytic and plasma cell reaction on the surface that is thought to be related to subsequent spontaneous deterioration of the valve structure (1).

Leakage of a prosthetic valve may occur at any time from hours to several years after implantation. Symptoms may develop gradually, with progressive fatigue and dyspnoea, or acutely with acute cardiac decompensation. Overall and operative mortality is related to the type of valve, the preoperative condition of the patient and the degree of urgency of operation.

With the exception of patients who can be electively operated upon, mitral valve reoperations have a consistently higher mortality than aortic valve reoperations. This is possibly because more mitral valve reoperations need to be done as emergencies. The overall mortality for elective reoperation is about 1.5%, for urgent reoperations 11% and for emergency reoperations 45% (2). I will restrict my discussion to the group of patients who need emergency surgery.

These patients are almost always unprepared and preoperative assessment often incomplete. Most will have clinical signs of circulatory failure if not frank cardiogenic shock. Especially when the mitral valve is involved, the pulmonary arterial pressure will be high, in some cases approaching systemic pressure, and these patients can present with acute pulmonary oedema. Some will require intubation and intermittent positive pressure ventilation before they reach the operating theatre. Providing anaesthesia for these patients can tax the resources of the most competent cardiac anaesthetist. Some of the important principles in the anaesthetic management of these patients will be discussed.

Premedication is seldom indicated or desirable - in the majority of patients consciousness will be sufficiently obtunded by diminished cerebral perfusion so that control of anxiety is relatively unimportant. Because of their critical haemodynamic status and reliance on vasoconstriction to maintain blood pressure, they are extremely sensitive to the cardiovascular depressant effects of sedative drugs. When cardiac catheterisation is carried out immediately before surgery, much valuable time will be saved if the cardiologist leaves a femoral arterial catheter in situ for subsequent arterial monitoring. It is often difficult to cannulate the radial artery in patients who are hypotensive and access to the femoral artery in the groin opposite that used for catheterisation should be reserved for introduction of an intra-aortic ballon catheter. IABP is often needed to wean these patients from cardiopulmonary bypass, and in the post-bypass period. Inotropic support should be continued during induction of anaesthesia and until bypass and is invariably needed for some time in the postbypass period. For near-moribund patients, some advocate instituting femoro-femoral bypass under local analgesia, with pump flows up to 2 l/min, sufficient to support the circulation during induction of anaesthesia. However this introduces delay and in my experience it is preferable to proceed immediately with anaesthesia, with the surgical team fully prepared.

There is no ideal technique of anaesthesia that can be universally used in this situation and the experience of the anaesthetist and his/her knowledge of the pharmacological properties of the drugs with which he/she is familiar is the most important factor. However a technique of anaesthesia should be chosen which fulfills the following requirements:

1) Does not cause depression of the myocardium
2) Has minimum effect on peripheral resistance
3) Has minimal effect on heart rate
4) Does not cause or exacerbate arrhythmias.

In general the barbiturates and inhalational anaesthetic agents should be avoided since they are cardiodepressant and reduce sympathetic activity. A small doses of diazepam (0.1-0.5 mg/kg) has been recommended for inducing anaesthesia in this emergency situation (3). The cardiovascular effects of intravenous diazepam are benign. It does not cause myocardial depression (4) and has no sympatholytic effects in man (5). My personal preference is to use fentanyl for induction and maintenance of anaesthesia. Fentanyl, 75 ug/kg, has minimal effects on myocardial function or haemodynamics in patients undergoing elective valvular surgery (6). However, in the emergency situation discussed here, the normal dose requirements must be reduced considerably. Often a total dose of 0.5 mg (10 ml) or less, which must be given slowly, will be sufficient to induce unconsciousness with minimum haemodynamic changes. For some anaesthetists ketamine, unique among anaesthetic drugs for its actions on the central nervous and cardiovascular systems, would be the drug of choice for induction of anaesthesia. It produces unconsciousness almost as rapidly as thiopentone (7) while maintaining or increasing sympathetic activity (8). Ketamine is therefore useful for induction of anaesthesia in patients dependent on sympathetic activity for maintenance of cardiovascular function. However, critically ill patients occasionally respond to ketamine with an unexpected drop in blood pressure which may result from the inability of the sympathomimetic actions of ketamine to counteract its direct myocardial depressant and vasodilatory effects (9).

The increase in systemic vascular resistance that may occur after ketamine may be detrimental to patients with acute valvular regurgitation, especially of the mitral valve, when the left atrium is of relatively normal size or is non-compliant. In this situation any increase in vascular resistance, by increasing impedance to ejection into the aorta, will increase regurgitation across the incompetent mitral valve. A 20 mmHg increase in MAP results in a 50% increase in left atrial pressure, a 120% rise in regurgitant flow and a 16% decrease in effective stroke volume (10). The same applies, though to a lesser degree, to aortic regurgitation. This suggests that vasodilator therapy with nitroprusside or nitroglycerine may be beneficial for these patients. Nitroprusside is of proven value in patients with mitral regurgitation secondary to papillary muscle dysfunction after myocardial infarction (11). In patients with acute aortic regurgitation with elevated left ventricular end diastolic pressure, nitroprusside reduces the regurgitant fraction and increases forward stroke volume (12). It is important however that diastolic pressure decreases are minimised otherwise myocardial blood supply will be further, and perhaps irreversibly, jeoparised. There is little information in the literature on the value of vasodilators in the management of patients with acute regurgitation due to prosthetic valve dysfunction. My own experience is that they are of value, if used with extreme caution, in patients with high systemic vascular resistance. The normally elevated resistance in these patients is frequently exacerbated by the high doses of inotropes required to maintain myocardial contractility and the judicious addition of nitroprusside will often improve forward cardiac output.

The problems of the anaesthetist do not cease with induction of anaesthesia and full attention must be given to maintaining circulatory support. During sternotomy there is an increased risk of complication, as with all reoperations, in these cases exacerbated by the emergency of the situation. In one study (2) involving 552 patients, 23 had complications during sternal reopening, including five patients where the right atrium was opened, seven patients with lacerations of the right ventricle, nine with aortic injury and in two patients previously placed aorta-coronary grafts were divided.

After bypass improvement in the conditions of the patient may be expected although some may need intensive support, including IABP, for some time postoperatively.

REFERENCES

1. Ferrans VJ, Spray TL, Billingham ME, Roberts WL: Structural changes in glutaraldehyde treated porcine heterografts used as substitute cardiac valves. Am. J. Cardiol. 41: 1159-1184, 1978.
2. Huseby DG, Pluth JR, Piehler JM, et al: Reoperation on prosthetic heart valves. An analysis of risk factors in 552 patients. J. Thorac. Cardiovasc. Surg. 86: 543-552, 1983.
3. Branthwaite MA: Anaesthesia for cardiac surgery and related procedures. Oxford, Blackwell Scientific Publications, p. 127, 1977.
4. D'Amelio G, Volta DS, Stritoni P, et al: Acute cardiovascular effects of diazepam in patients with mitral valve disease. Eur. J. Clin. Pharmacol. 6: 61-63, 1973.
5. Bradshaw EG: The vasodilator effects of diazepam in vitro. Br. J. Anaesth. 48: 817-818, 1976.
6. Bovill JG, Warren PJ, Schuller JL, van Wezel HB, Hoeneveld MH: Comparison of fentanyl, sufentanil and alfentanil anesthesia in patients undergoing valvular heart surgery. Anesth. Analg. 63: 1081-1086, 1984.
7. Bovill JG, Coppel DL, Dundee JW, Moore J: Current status of ketamine anaesthesia. Lancet 1: 1285-1288, 1971.
8. Traber DL, Wilson RD: Involvement of the sympathetic nervous system in the pressor response to ketamine. Anesth. Analg. 48: 248-252, 1969.
9. Waxman K, Shoemaker WC, Lippmann M: Cardiovascular effects of anesthetic induction with ketamine. Anesth. Analg. 59: 355-358, 1980.
10. Jose AD, Taylor RR, Bernstein L: The influence of arterial pressure on mitral incompetence in man. J. Clin. Invest. 43: 2094, 1964.
11. Chatterjee K, Parmley WA, Swan HJC, et al: Beneficial effects of vasodilator agents in severe mitral regurgitation due to dysfunction of subvalvular apparatus. Circulation 48: 684-690, 1973.
12. Miller RR, Vismara LA, DeMaria AN, et al: Afterload reduction therapy with nitroprusside in severe aortic regurgitation: Improved cardiac performance and reduced regurgitant volume. Am. J. Cardiol. 38: 564-567, 1976.

MASSIVE PULMONARY EMBOLISM

Peter J.A. van der Starre, M.D.

INTRODUCTION

Massive pulmonary embolism is not such a rare condition as is often reported. Since most of the cases have a lethal outcome, only a few reports have been published concerning the acute surgical treatment of patients with this clinical syndrome (1,2). A case report is presented from which a few conclusions can be made.

CASE REPORT

A 41 years old woman, who had a caesarean section 14 days before admission, giving birth to a premature child. She had a history of smoking, and of thrombosis 4 years earlier, without any serious sequalae. She was admitted to a local hospital in a serious condition, with dyspnoea, arrythmias and hypotension. This condition developed within a few hours, from which the refering cardiologist made the diagnosis of pulmonary embolism. A quickly-performed arteriogram of the pulmonary artery showed a complete stop in the right pulmonary artery, and a low flow state of the left pulmonary artery (fig. 1).

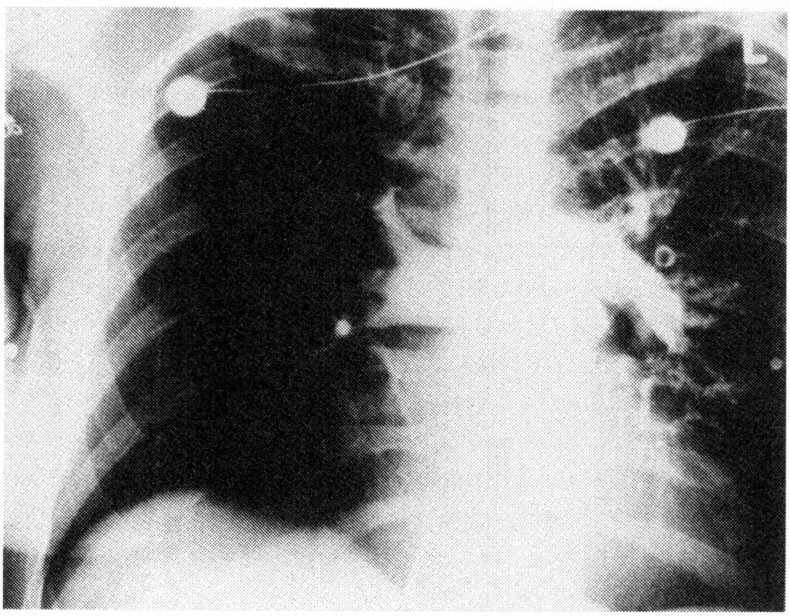

Figure 1: preoperative angiography, showing total occlusion of the right pulmonary artery.

The patient was transported to the cardiac surgical clinic, where she was in a disastrous state at admission. She was already intubated because of a low PO_2, (55 mmHg), developed arrythmias, for which lidocaine was injected, and hypotension (blood pressure 60/30 mmHg). She was oliguric for 12 hours and had a temperature of 34.8°C. A pre-operative bloodgas analysis showed a metabolic acidosis with a base-excess of minus 7. The ECG (fig. 2) showed a right ventricular strain, and an axis shift to the right.

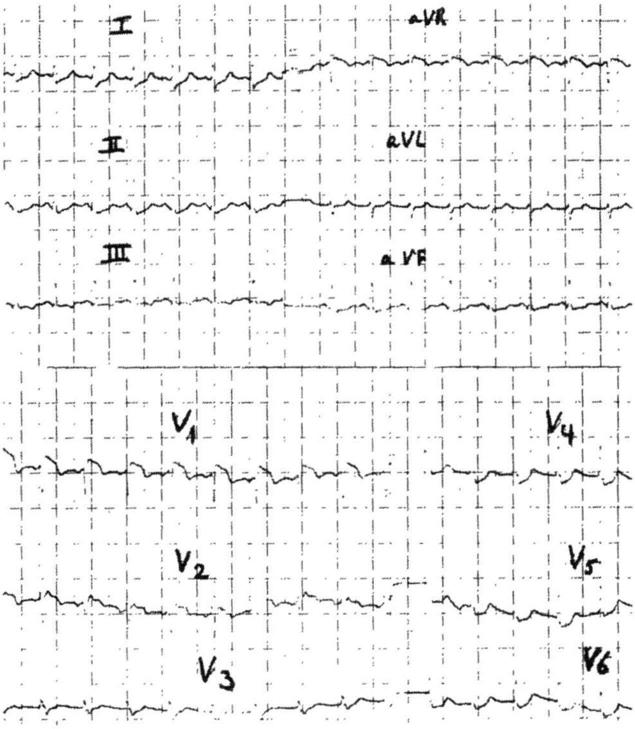

Figure 2: preoperative E.C.G., showing strain of the right ventricle and axis-shift.

Induction of anesthesia was performed using etomidate, fentanyl and pancuronium with 100% oxygen ventilation. The condition of the patient did not deteriorate before cardiopulmonary bypass. Dopamine was started before induction 6 microgr/kg/min (to keep systolic blood pressure ± 90 mmHg). Monitoring consisted of continuous intra-arterial blood pressure monitoring, ECG and heart rate, and an introducer was inserted in the right internal jugular vein to monitor central venous pressure, and to have an access route for inserting a Swan Ganz catheter postoperatively. After starting cardiopulmonary bypass, the patient was cooled to 23°C (nasopharyngeal), followed by stopping the heart using a hypokalemic cardioplegic solution. When the pulmonary artery was opened, large clots were removed from the right and left pulmonary artery, and from the right ventricle. After opening the right atrium there appeared to be large clots in both caval veins as well. The right ventricle appeared to be dilated, but no signs of infarction could be detected. After closure of the heart and the pulmonary artery the patient was rewarmed and weaned from bypass successfully. Just before decannulation of the venous

cannula, a low output syndrome developed with hypotension, dilatation of the right atrium and right ventricle. Complete cardiopulmonary bypass was re-instituted, and the right atrium was re-opened. Again large clots were removed from the right ventricle and the right atrium, and also the inferior vena cava. After reclosure of the heart, the patients was once more weaned of bypass uneventfully, with the use of dopamine 6 microgr/kg/min to increase blood pressure. Immediately postoperatively the decision was made to insert a Swan Ganz catheter to monitor the pulmonary artery pressure, because of the peroperative observation that the right ventricle was severely dilated. After insertion of the thermodilution catheter, pulmonary artery pressure (PAP) appeared to be 46/29 mmHg, central venous pressure (CVP 12 mmHg and pulmonary capillary wedge pressure (PCWP) 5 mmHg. Blood pressure was 95/65 mmHg, and cardiac index (CI) 1.7 $l/m^2/min$, for which reason dobutamine was added to the dopamine at a dose of 4 microgr/kg/min. CI increased to 2,1 $l/m^2/min$, and blood pressure to 120/60 mmHg. Because PAP remained high, ketanserin 0,2 mg/kg/hr was started to decrease pulmonary vascular resistance. The patient was transfered to the intensive care unit, but unfortunately developed signs of tamponade in the evening. It has to be mentioned that a heparin-infusion (20.000 units/24 hours) was started postoperatively, to keep APTT between 60 and 80 seconds. The patient underwent a rethoracotomy, revealing a large blood clot in front of the heart and $\pm$ 400 cc of free blood around the heart. The procedure went uneventfully, and the patient was transfered to the ICU.
The following day PAP decreased to 28/15 mmHg, CVP to 6 mmHg and PCWP remained 5 mmHg. CI increased to 2,5 $l/m^2/min$. As soon as oral feeding was possible, coumarine derivatives were started and heparin was terminated. The hospital course went uneventful during 14 days, and the patient went home in a good clinical condition. The ECG in that period appeared to be completely normal (fig. 3).

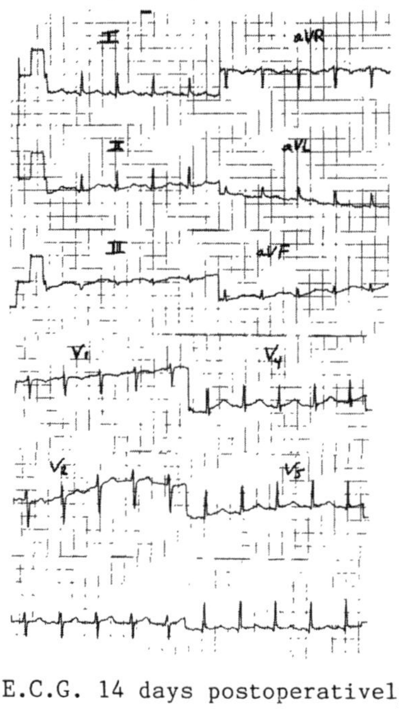

Figure 3: E.C.G. 14 days postoperatively. No abnormalities.

DISCUSSION

Acute pulmonary embolism is a common clinical entity occuring in over ..00.000 symptomatic episodes each year in the United States (3). Only a few of these cases are admitted for surgery, with a high mortality rate. Concerning the etiology of thrombosis and emboli, the classical triad of Virchow, consisting of vascular stasis, vessel wall damage and coaguability changes is still valid. The most important sources for emboli are the deep veins of the legs, and pelvic veins from the ileofemoral and renal tract (4). Predisposing factors are listed in table 1, but it has to be mentioned that this listing is certainly not complete (5).

Trauma surgery
Immobility
Pregnancy
Old age
Adiposistas
Varicosis
Malignancy
Myeloproliterative syndromes
Gram-negative sepsis
Oestrogenic agents

TABLE 1: Predisposing factors for venous thrombosis and embolism

Generally speaking the management of pulmonary emboli without serious circulatory impairment, consists of the use of anticoagulants like heparin, urokinase or streptokinase, and the treatment of the coexisting pulmonary hypertension (6).

The surgical approach is especially necessary when the patient develops acute pulmonary emboli with circulatory failure, since the mortality of the medical treatment of this syndrome is almost 100%. The clinical manifenstation of acute pulmonary embolism is mostly hypotension, dyspnoea, sometimes syncope and sweating (7). The patients shows an intense vasoconstriction, with high venous pressures. As in our case report the ECG shows a right ventricular strain, sometimes with T-wave inversion and axis shift. The diagnosis is confirmed by arteriography of the pulmonary artery, which should be done as soon as possible. The surgical interference consists of connecting the patient as quickly as possible on cardiopulmonary bypass, opening the pulmonary artery and removing the clots, and if recurrence is expected, a ligation, partial ligation or filtering of the inferior vena cava has to be considered (1,2).

From the anesthetic point of view the most important feature of the anesthesia regimen should be the avoidance of the use of negative inotropic agents and the prevention of a further increase of the pulmonary vascular resistance, which is generally high (10). This means that nitrous oxide for example should not be used (8). Before induction one has to consider starting a dopmaine of dobutamine infusion to support the circulation during the procedure before bypass, since most of the induction agents cause a peripheral vasodilatation, which can be deleterious in these patients with an already low cardiac output (11). In our hands the choice of the anesthetic technique consists mainly of the use of analgesic agents like fentanyl, sufentanil, an induction agent

with minimal circulatory influence (etomidate), and a muscle relaxant which does not cause peripheral vasodilatation (pancuronium, vecuronium). The patient is ventilated with 100% oxygen, because usually hypoxia exists (9). In the postoperative management the support of the circulation by using positive inotropic agents and pulmonary vasodilators (nitroglycerin, nitroprussid, ketanserin) is recommended (12), and it depends on the ventilatory progression whether the patient should be ventilated mechanically for a longer period or not (9).
In view of monitoring, the use of a thermodilution pulmonary artery catheter pre-operatively is debatable, although no reports are presented concerning this item. Our choice was to insert a pulmonary artery catheter postoperatively, to be able to titrate positive inotropic agents like dopamine and dobutamine according to the calculated cardiac output and pulmonary and systemic vascular resistance (10).

REFERENCES

1. Greenfiled LJ. Pulmonary embolism: pathophysiology and treatment. In: Thoracic and Cardiovascular Surgery. Ed. Glenn WWL. Norvalik, Appleton-Century-Crofts, 1983, pp 1284-1286
2. Bomalaski JS, Marten GJ, Hughes RL. Inferior vena cava interruption in the management of pulmonary embolis. Chest 1982;82:767-773
3. Dalen JE, Alpert JS. Natural history of pulmonary embolism. Prog. Cardiovasc. Dis. 1975;17:259-270
4. Byrne JJ, O'Neil EE. Fatal pulmonary emboli: A study of 130 autopsy proven fatal emboli: Am. J. Surg. 1952;83:47-60
5. Coon WW. Epidemiology of venous thromboembolism. Ann. Surg. 1977;186:149-164
6. National Cooperative Study. The urokinase-pulmonary embolism trial. Circulation 1973;47:suppl II
7. Bell WR, Simon TL, Demets DL. The clinical features of submassive and massive pulmonary emboli. Am. J. Med. 1977;62:355-370
8. Hildenberg JC, McCammon RL, Stoelting RK. Pulmonary and systemic vascular responses to nitrous oxide in patients with stenosis and pulmonary hypertension. Anesth. Analg. 1980;59:323-326
9. D'Alonzo GE, Bower JS, De Hart P. The mechanisms of abnormal gas exchange in acute massive pulmonary embolism. An. Rev. Respir. Dis. 1983;128:170-175
10. Brown DL, Bodary AK, Kirby RR. Anesthetic management of pulmonary thromboendarterectomy. Anesthesiology 1984;61:197-200
11. Stool EW, Mullims CB, Leshin SJ, Mitchell JH. Dimensional changes of the left ventricle during acute pulmonary arterial hypertension in dogs. Am. J. Cardiol. 1974;33:868-875
12. Rosenthal MH, Pearl RG, Schroeder JS, Ashton JPA. Nitroglycerin versus nitroprusside in pulmonary hypertension. Anesthesiology 1981;55:A79

RUPTURED CORONARY ARTERY FOLLOWING ANGIOPLASTY

Norbert P. de Bruijn, M.D., Fiona M. Clements, M.D.

Although percutaneous transluminal coronary angioplasty (PTCA) appears to be a relatively safe procedure, reported complications include coronary occlusion and dissection with or without myocardial infarction. Coronary rupture is a very infrequent complication of PTCA, there being only one case in 3,079 patients enrolled in the NHLBI PTCA Registry. The case reported in the literature[1] regarded a 77 year old man with unstable angina pectoris with focal severe stenosis of a dominant right coronary artery. PTCA of the right coronary artery was performed. After an initially successful dilatation, coronary angiography three months later disclosed significant stenosis again at the same site. Repeat PTCA was performed. Multiple inflations of a 3 mm. catheter at a manual pressure of 9 atmospheres dilated the stenosis to about a 60% occlusive lesion. A 3.7 mm. catheter was subsequently positioned and inflated five times at the maximal pressure of ten atmospheres. On the fifth inflation the proximal end of the balloon ruptured. Angiography demonstrated extravasation of contrast material into the epicardial tissue plus runoff into the distal right coronary artery. The heart rate and arterial blood pressure quickly decreased, blood was drained from the pericardial sac, but fatal cardiac arrest ensued. At necropsy an elliptical rupture site measuring 0.6 cm. in the long axis was present in the right coronary artery.

In a recent publication acute coronary events associated with percutaneous transluminal coronary angioplasty were reported[2]. Data on 3,079 patients in the NHLBI PTCA Registry were reported from 105 contributing centers. Coronary vascular events (dissection, occlusion, spasm, embolism, perforation or rupture) or ischemic events (MI or prolonged angina) occurred in 418 patients (13.6%). Major complications (MI, emergency surgery or death) occurred in 280 patients (67%) with acute coronary events. Death occurred in 29 patients (0.9%), nonfatal MI in 154 (5.0%). An emergency CABG without death or infarction in 106 (3.4%).

The recent introduction of a perfusion catheter consisting of a long distal segment with multiple sideholes which can be advanced over the guidewire once coronary dissection or occlusion has occurred has greatly enhanced the successful management of patients with acute coronary events undergoing emergency coronary artery bypass grafting. The continued perfusion of the myocardium distal to the occluded coronary artery has basically provided circumstances which are similar to those in patients undergoing elective coronary artery bypass surgery. Not only will the perfusion catheter ensure the continued perfusion of endangered myocardium, but it will allow the delivery of cardioplegic solution to the myocardium at risk, thus increasing the chance of a favorable outcome.

The anesthetic considerations in patients referred for emergency coronary artery bypass grafting following failed PTCA or PTCA complicated by coronary occlusion due to dissection, spasm, perforation or rupture are fairly straightforward. Because these patients are in the process of developing a myocardial infarction, speed is a very important consideration. If the cooperation between the interventional cardiologist, the surgeon and the anesthesiologist is optimal, early warning should have been given and there will be ample time to set up the operating room before the patient arrives. The anesthesiologist should go to the cardiac catheterization laboratory, assess the patient and judge whether temporary therapeutic interventions in the form of intravenous nitrotriglycerine, sublingual nifedipine, prophylactic lidocaine and intravenous morphine are indicated and have been instituted and if satisfied organize for the patient to be taken to the operating room as soon as possible. The arterial sheath introduced by the cardiologist should not be removed because it may be used to measure arterial pressure in the operating room. If insertion of an intraaortic counterpulsation balloon would add substantial delay in proceeding with the surgery it is our practice not to insert one, but to proceed to the operating room immediately. Upon arrival in the operating room we use the arterial sheath to measure systemic arterial pressure, establish a large bore venous cannula and proceed with the induction of anesthesia. In these patients we do not insert a pulmonary artery catheter before induction of anesthesia because we feel that the additional stress would be detrimental. We consider these patients to have a full stomach and take the appropriate cautionary measures to prevent aspiration. After induction of anesthesia while the patient is being prepped a pulmonary artery catheter is inserted. After induction of anesthesia these patients most often seem to become more stable and recently we have felt comfortable enough to allow the surgeons to take down an internal mammary artery before instituting cardiopulmonary bypass. This is especially true if the cardiologists have been able to pass a perfusion catheter through the lesion so that some coronary flow is still present.

In those patients who have received either intravenous or intracoronary doses of streptokinase we administer epsilon amino caproic acid in an early stage of the operation in order to have normal coagulation after discontinuation of cardiopulmonary bypass.

References:

1) Saffitz JE, Rose TE, Oakes JB, et al. Coronary Arterial Rupture During Coronary Angioplasty. Am.J.Cardiol. 51:902-904, 1983.

2) Cowley MJ, Dorros G, Kelsey SF, et al. Acute Coronary Events Associated With Percutaneous Transluminal Coronary Angioplasty. Am.J.Cardiol. 53:12C-16C, 1984.

INDEX

GPSR Compliance
The European Union's (EU) General Product Safety Regulation (GPSR) is a set of rules that requires consumer products to be safe and our obligations to ensure this.

If you have any concerns about our products, you can contact us on

ProductSafety@springernature.com

In case Publisher is established outside the EU, the EU authorized representative is:

Springer Nature Customer Service Center GmbH
Europaplatz 3
69115 Heidelberg, Germany

www.ingramcontent.com/pod-product-compliance
Ingram Content Group UK Ltd.
Pitfield, Milton Keynes, MK11 3LW, UK
UKHW020815290926
15470UKWH00003B/1167
* 9 7 8 0 8 9 8 3 8 7 9 4 0 *